Healing Yourself with Self-Hypnosis

Revised by Dr. Caroline Miller,
American Institute of Hypnotherapy

Frank Caprio, M.D. and Joseph R. Berger

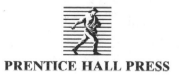

PRENTICE HALL PRESS

Library of Congress Cataloging-in-Publication Data

Caprio, Frank Samuel.
     Healing yourself with self-hypnosis / Frank Caprio and Joseph R. Berger ;
revised by Caroline Miller. — Rev. and expanded ed.
     p. cm.
     Includes index.
     ISBN 0-13-906678-0 (case). — ISBN 0-7352-0004-1 (paper)
     1. Health. 2. Autogenic training. 3. Mind and body. I. Berger, Joseph R.
II. Miller, Caroline. III. Title.
RA776.5.C363 1998   97-53295
615.8'512—dc21   CIP

Acquisitions Editor: *Doug Corcoran*
Production Editor: *Sharon L. Gonzalez*
Formatting/Interior Design: *Robyn Beckerman*

The information presented in this book is designed to help you make informed decisions about your health. It is not intended as a substitute for medical care nor a manual for self-treatment. If you feel that you have a medical problem, seek professional medical advice promptly.

Printed in the United States of America

10 9 8 7 6 5 4 3 2

ISBN 0-7352-0004-1 (p)

 PRENTICE HALL PRESS
Paramus, NJ 07652

A Simon & Schuster Company

On the World Wide Web at http://www.phdirect.com

Prentice Hall International (UK) Limited, *London*
Prentice Hall of Australia Pty. Limited, *Sydney*
Prentice Hall Canada, Inc., *Toronto*
Prentice Hall Hispanoamericana, S.A., *Mexico*
Prentice Hall of India Private Limited, *New Delhi*
Prentice Hall of Japan, Inc., *Tokyo*
Simon & Schuster Asia Pte. Ltd., *Singapore*
Editora Prentice Hall do Brasil, Ltda., *Rio de Janeiro*

To Joe and John
Jill and Aaron
Zack and Zane
You're the best

It matters not how strait the gate,
How charged with punishment the scroll,
I am the master of my fate;
I am the captain of my soul.

—WILLIAM ERNEST HENLEY

Acknowledgments

I want to thank the people who have shared their knowledge and experiences with me over the years—my mentors, my teachers, and my students. You have taught me and demonstrated to me that we can indeed change our lives in remarkable ways. You've shown me that the human mind is an awesome thing, capable of stunning achievements.

I am grateful to my colleagues at the American Institute of Hypnotherapy for their amazing support and constant collaboration as we continue to learn more about this fascinating art and science of hypnosis. Special appreciation goes to my extraordinary associate (accomplice?), AIH General Counsel Robert Strouse, JD. Bob is a walking dichotomy: intelligent, witty, and compassionate business-man—all in the body of an attorney! Thanks for making AIH such a pleasurable place to work.

My gratitude also extends to my family, who were all so supportive of this project: my husband Joseph and my sons Joe and John.

I wish to acknowledge the work of Dr. Frank Caprio and Mr. Joseph Berger, whose efforts helped so many thousands of people. Their research and techniques made a significant contribution to the body of knowledge of this field.

Finally, I thank Mr. Douglas Corcoran, senior editor at Prentice Hall, for giving me the opportunity to participate in this rewarding project. Working with you has been a pleasure.

Contents

INTRODUCTION

Self-Hypnosis: The New Way to Successful Living—1

Better Health, More Happiness, Greater Success
   Are Attainable Goals 1
How This Book Came About 2
The Purpose of This Book 2
What Self-Hypnosis Can Do 2
All Hypnosis Is Self-Hypnosis 3
Self-Hypnosis Gives You Unlimited Potential 3
Self Hypnosis Enables You to Discover and Develop
   Your New Self 6
You Can Enjoy Better Health Through Self-Hypnosis 7
Self-Hypnosis Will Help You Achieve Personality Maturity 7
Successful Planning 8
Self-Hypnosis Can Improve Your Love Life 9
How to Use This Book to Your Greatest Advantage 10

CHAPTER 1

Hypnosis: Theories, Fallacies, and Facts—11

Everyone Has Been Hypnotized 11
Definition of Hypnosis 11
Origin of the Word 12

There Are Two Kinds of Hypnosis 12
What Is Meant by the Hypnotic State? 13
Theories of Hypnosis. 13
Common Fallacies and Facts. 14
Hypnosis Versus Self-Hypnosis 18
Self-Hypnosis in Our Daily Lives. 19
Hypnosis and Self-Hypnosis: Forces for Good 20
Self-Hypnosis Works Automatically 21

CHAPTER 2

How and Why Hypnosis Works—23

Different Ways in Which We Receive Suggestions 24
The Power of Your Early Conditioning 26
The Conditioned-Reflex Response. 28
We Behave Like Trained Animals 28
Emotion: The Most Important Element. 29
Conditioned Responses You May Know Very Well 30
The Good News 31
Find Out for Yourself. 31
All Hypnosis Is Self-Hypnosis: The Discovery. 32

CHAPTER 3

Boosting Your Brain Power—35

The Miracle of the Human Body. 35
Your Amazing Brain. 36
Left Brain, Right Brain 37
Left Hemisphere 37
Right Hemisphere 38
Two Ways of Knowing. 38
Why We Don't Use Both Sides of Our Brain. 41

Determining Your Own Dominant Hemisphere. 41
The New Era of the Mind. 49
Moving into the New Millennium 49

CHAPTER 4

Your Mind: Conscious and Subconscious—51

Self-Hypnosis Can Release Hidden Potential Within You 51
Your Mind Is More Than a Brain. 52
How Your Mind Processes Information 52
Your Conscious and Subconscious Minds at Work. 53
Your Conscious Mind. 53
Your Subconscious Mind 54
Your Motivation Determines Your Results. 57
Increasing Your Motivation. 57
Study Your Dreams—They Can Tell You Much About
     Your Subconscious Self 58
How to Make Your Subconscious Mind Work for You. 59
What You Think About, You Become 62
The Choice Is Yours 63
Words Are Important 63
Using Words That Work: Setting S.M.A.R.T. Goals 64

CHAPTER 5

The 4-A's Method of Self-Hypnosis: A Step-by-Step Plan—67

First Decide What You Want Self-Hypnosis to Do for You 68
The 4-A's Method of Self-Hypnosis 69
How to Achieve Self-Hypnosis in the Waking State. 76
How to Rouse Yourself out of the Hypnotic State. 76
Always Keep This in Mind 76
A Word of Caution 77

Regarding Emotional Problems 77
An Added Advantage: The Experience of Being Hypnotized 78
How You Can Most Effectively Use This Book 79
Work on One Thing at a Time 80
A World of "Shoulds" and Sabotage. 80
Remember the Power of Past Suggestions 81
Take Responsibility for Your Life. 81

CHAPTER 6

Making a Plan: The First Step to Success—83

Begin Your Planning 83
Make a List. 84
Are Your Feelings Showing? 85
The Advantages of Intelligent Planning 86
Does This Sound Familiar? 86
Making a Plan Makes a Difference: Autoanalysis Can Help 87

CHAPTER 7

The Amazing Power of Self-Hypnosis
for Daily Health and Weight Control—89

Establishing Good Health Habits with Self-Hypnosis 89
Daily Health Reminders 89
Self-Hypnosis: The Modern Approach to Successful
    Weight Control 91
Overeating Is a Form of "Psychic Suicide" 92
The Power of Suggestion—Again! 92
Lose the "Diet" Mentality 93
The Emotional Issue of Weight 93
Calories *Do* Count. . . . However 94

A Nine-Step Program for Weight Reduction 94
What Losing Weight the Self-Hypnosis Way Will Do for You 98
You Have the Power 103

CHAPTER 8

Self-Hypnosis, Smoking, Alcohol, and Drugs—105

Facts About Smoking: The Bad News. 105
Facts About Not Smoking: The Good News 106
Smoking: It's Just a Habit 107
Why Did You Start? 108
Suggestions to Follow if You Want to Stop Smoking 108
The Problem of Alcoholism and Other Addictions. 112
Subconscious Causes of Excessive Drinking 112
The Treatment of Alcoholism 114
Self Hypnosis Can Help 114
Drug Addiction 116
Addictions and Addictive Thinking 116
Self-Hypnosis and Drugs 117
What Does It Take to Quit?. 117
Suggestions That Will Assist You in Designing
    Your Personalized Program. 118

CHAPTER 9

The Hypnotic Road to Restful Sleep—121

How Much Sleep Is Enough?. 121
Many Factors Cause Sleeplessness 122
How to Induce Restful Sleep. 125
Some Self-Hypnotic Exercises for Restful Sleep 125
Self-Hypnosis Leads You to Sleep Naturally 126

CHAPTER 10

What Self-Hypnosis Can Do to Make Your Sex Life More Exciting—127

Self-Love: The Most Important Element 128
Avoidance of Sex. 128
The Use of Self-Hypnosis for the Problem of Impotence 131
Start with an Inventory of Your Sex Life. 133
Questions to Ask Yourself. 134
Twenty-one Suggestions to Give Yourself in Autotherapy. 134

CHAPTER 11

Overcome Tension, Chronic Tiredness, and Pain with Self-Hypnosis—137

Attitudes Are Habitual 139
Tension Becomes a Habit. 139
Tension Breeds Psychosomatic Difficulties 140
Tension Breeds Fatigue 140
Is Your Work "Working" for You?. 141
Own Your Attitudes and Habits. 141
A Feeling Analyzed Is a Feeling Owned. 142
Self-Hypnosis: Your Built-in Tranquilizer 142
The Worry Habit: What Can You Do?. 143
Twenty-five Examples of Self-Suggestions for Attitudes, Feelings,
    and Worry. 144
Develop a Sense of Humor: It's a Great Tension Reducer! 145
Hypnosis and Pain Control: It's Nothing New 146
Pain Serves a Purpose 146
How We "Make It All Better" for Little Children 147
Removing the Feeling of Pain 147
Some Imagery for Pain Control 148

The Posthypnotic Suggestion Is Important 149
Ten Posthypnotic Suggestions for Pain Control 150
A Final Word. 150

CHAPTER 12
Master Your Emotions Through Self-Hypnosis—151

Triumph over Your Fears with Self-Hypnosis 151
Is Fear at Fault? 153
Ten General Self-Suggestions for Fear 153
Self-Hypnosis Can Help You Conquer Anger 154
How to Overcome the Fear of Flying with Self-Hypnosis 159

CHAPTER 13
You Can Defeat Mental Depression and Unhappy Moods with Self-Hypnosis—165

Analyze the Nature and Cause of Your Unhappy Moods 165
What You Should Know About Mental Depression 166
Use Posthypnotic Suggestion to Divert Your Mind from Yourself. 168
Twenty Self-Hypnotic Suggestions for Banishing the Blues. 171

CHAPTER 14
How to Create for Yourself a New Personality and a Happier Life—173

What Is Meant by "Personality"? 173
What Made You What You Are 174
Can You Change Your Personality? 175
The Self-Hypnosis Approach to Personality Change. 176

How to Acquire a Magnetic Personality 178
Ten Posthypnotic Suggestions to Give Yourself for Getting Along
    with Others. 179
Develop a Tolerant Personality with Self-Hypnosis 180
Enlist the Cooperation of Your Friends for Personality Improvement . . 181
Self-Hypnosis Improves Your Memory and Ability to Learn 183
Fifteen Self-Suggestions for Learning and Memory Improvement. 184
Self-Hypnosis for Concentration and Study 185

CHAPTER 15

How to Achieve Hypnotic Power for Yourself and Influence over Others—189

What Getting Along with People by Using Self-Hypnosis
    Can Do for You. 190
Self-Hypnosis Enhances Sales Ability 191
Visual Reminders. 193
Twenty Self-Suggestions for Increasing Your Hypnotic Power
    and Appeal. 194

CHAPTER 16

Using Hypnotic Magic to Stay Young and Live Longer—195

You Are As Old As You Feel. 195
Make Happier Living Your Goal 195
A Theory of Aging: Mind over Body 196
Let Your Work Become Your Hobby 199
Hypnosis and Religion 200
Self-Hypnosis Makes Prayer More Effective. 201
I Believe. 203
What to Remember 204

CHAPTER 17

Richer Living Through New Thought Patterns—205

You and Heredity 207
Making the Most of Each Day 208
Twenty-five Guaranteed Dividends 210
A Reinforced Suggestion 212

CHAPTER 18

Questions and Answers About Self-Hypnosis—213

Epilogue—223

APPENDIX 1

*The Best Autorelaxation/Induction Procedures
for You to Hypnotize Yourself—225*

APPENDIX 2

Exercises in Imagery and Awareness—243

APPENDIX 3

Self-Hypnosis Therapeutic Suggestions—253

References—265

Index—267

Self-Hypnosis: The New Way to Successful Living

Self-hypnosis can bring great benefits to your life—more energy, better health, lasting peace of mind, success, and happiness.

Better Health, More Happiness, Greater Success Are Attainable Goals

The pursuit of health, happiness, and success is a universal goal. Everyone would like to enjoy good health. Everyone wants to be happy. Everyone wants to experience the satisfaction of a successful life.

We are of the opinion that, given the proper knowledge and guidance, anyone who has a sincere desire for better health, improved relationships, more success, and, in general, a happier life can do so. This book is designed to provide you with detailed explanations of how to develop your personal capacity for self-hypnosis.

This is not a book on psychiatry for the nonprofessional. We have instead focused on the importance of correct thinking. It is our intent to show you how the mind influences every specter of your life. We will teach what you can do to achieve inner strength, survive adversities, and improve yourself in ways that will assist you in leading a fuller, richer life.

1

All of us have greater mind power than we realize. Everything within reason is humanly possible. We need never consider ourselves failures or remain unhappy. There is always much that we can do to correct and improve our situation in life.

How This Book Came About

The book was originally inspired by the public's response to an article, "Think Your Fears Away," that was published by *The American Weekly*, January 31, 1960. From the letters we received, we knew that there must be thousands of people looking for guidance as to how they can help themselves, how they can improve themselves and achieve a fuller, richer life.

The Purpose of This Book

Our purpose in writing this book is to convince you—by having you prove it to yourself—that self-hypnosis can do for you the things you want it to do. It can be a tremendous weapon at your command, enabling you to manage everyday situations with mastery.

That your mind is the MASTER OF YOUR LIFE is the basic message of this book. It is founded on the proven philosophy that TO LIVE RIGHT YOU MUST THINK RIGHT. *How you live is how you use your mind.*

What Self-Hypnosis Can Do

Soon you will see what self-hypnosis can do for you in using the vast potential of your mind to reshape your reality. You can develop your memory, creativity, and public-speaking ability. You can transform nervousness into helpful, productive energy. You can eliminate unwanted habits and control your weight. Fears can be reduced or eliminated and a positive self-image cultivated. You can remember where you misplaced an object or ease yourself to sleep more easily at night. You can prepare for surgery or the birth of a child. You can attract more love and find more fulfillment in life. There is almost no limit to what you can do.

All Hypnosis Is Self-Hypnosis

We have engaged in many years of research with actual patients, and we know what can be accomplished with hypnosis. It is our belief that since all hypnosis is self-hypnosis, the average person can be taught the techniques of self-hypnosis to achieve most any accomplishment of his or her choosing.

Self-Hypnosis Gives You Unlimited Potential

Because hypnosis has somehow been historically surrounded by an aura of mysticism, it has always provided journalistic capital for all forms of media, from the performers of vaudeville shows early in the century to the vast electronic communications of today. Throughout the years, an immense amount of misinformation about hypnosis has been circulated and perpetuated. As a result, the general public does not have a true picture of the art and science of hypnosis. Many great achievements in the past have come about through hypnosis. However, only in recent years has it begun to come out of the dark age in which it was considered the work of the devil or a ridiculous stage act. It is no longer regarded as black magic. Hypnosis today has gained respect, dignity, and worldwide interest, holding a recognized place in behavioral science and medicine.

Hypnosis can be traced back as far as the era of primitive healers. However, self-hypnosis is a relatively new phenomenon.

Because human beings are so autosuggestible, self-hypnosis can do wonderful things. You can make your subconscious mind work to your advantage. Your subconscious mind plays a far more important role in your daily life than you probably realize.

"Self-hypnosis plays a valuable role in a process which makes it easier for an individual to discover and understand the workings of his own body and mind, learn the factors which basically cause his own distress and learn how to control them." This is how the late

Dr. Milton Erickson, probably the greatest medical hypnotherapist of the century, described the phenomenon of self-hypnosis.

Too many people today rely entirely on pills to relax them—pharmaceutical relaxation. We do not minimize the value that certain drugs have in specific cases where drug therapy is appropriate. However, we discourage the indiscriminate use of drugs when autorelaxation through self-hypnosis can be achieved so easily.

A FEW EXAMPLES OF WHAT SELF-HYPNOSIS
HAS BEEN ABLE TO DO:

An artist who loved to paint, but who lacked self-confidence, became a prizewinner several times over after learning the technique of self-hypnosis.

A once-successful writer, convinced that she was all washed up, was trained to relax while she wrote and to look more deeply into herself for the right words. She has since written three best-sellers.

An architect was taught to put himself in a self-hypnotic state for five minutes during which time he instructed his subconscious to produce for him, say, "ten different elevations" for the home he was designing.

A musician learned to get her subconscious mind to produce for her a new melody or a novel arrangement whenever she chose to use self-hypnosis.

A research scientist accelerated the creative process within himself to discover an astounding new theory.

A trial attorney learned to use hypnosis to enable him to use instant recall for the precedents he needed as he presented his case in court.

A well-known public figure who suffered acute anxiety when he had to address a group was taught self-hypnosis, and he was able to speak without fear.

Many children and adolescents have learned self-hypnosis to control their thought processes before they grow up to be anxiety-laden grownups!

We know that these things may sound fantastic, and we agree that they are. However, they represent just a fraction of the applications to creativity that we have witnessed for ourselves.

As we study the biographies of many of the genius minds of the past, we may easily infer that the spontaneous and unexplained phenomenon behind their superior abilities was simply self-hypnosis. Multiple references are made to a special state of consciousness variously referred to as trance, waking dream, ecstasy, super-normal feelings, and the like. Self-hypnosis may also be the secret behind some of our great scientists and inventors as well as financial geniuses.

FAMOUS PEOPLE WHO HAVE USED SELF-HYPNOSIS:

The great poet Tennyson was one. Many times he told how he would walk into the quiet of the woods and repeat his own name over and over to himself. This would cause him to feel transported into a new state of consciousness in which colors were more vivid and sounds more ethereal—a state in which words, phrases, sentences, and verses just came to him—and that he thereafter had only to copy them onto paper.

It is common knowledge that Mozart would often go for a ride in a coach and, while thus relaxing, hear the melodies and orchestrations that ultimately became his masterworks. Such a spontaneous auditory hallucination can most easily come to someone trained in self-hypnosis.

George Washington Carver, the great scientist, said, "All my life, I have risen regularly at four o'clock and have gone into the woods and talked with God. There He gives me my orders for the day . . ."

Thomas Edison believed that his inventions came to him from the "infinite forces in the universe," and that they came most readily when he was relaxed.

Henry Ford went into the solitude of his meditating room to solve problems and prepare his business plans.

In his book *Think and Grow Rich*, Napoleon Hill talked about his daily hallucinatory "meeting" with nine great individuals (Emerson, Paine, Edison, Darwin, Lincoln, Burbank, Napoleon, Ford, and Carnegie), his "invisible counselors."

Solitude, meditation, relaxation, talking with God or imaginary counselors are all different forms of the same thing—self-hypnosis.

We could almost endlessly cite such examples from history that demonstrate that artists, scientists, inventors, and business giants used the "natural gift" of self-hypnosis for the purpose of elevating themselves above the standard levels of achievement. Those individuals somehow had an intuitive knowledge about the trance state.

Now we know, however, that it is possible to teach this invaluable skill to anyone who wants to learn it. We know for a fact that you can learn to use hypnosis to change your life!

Self-Hypnosis Enables You to Discover and Develop Your New Self

You will begin to believe in yourself, acquire confidence you never had before. For the first time in your life you will experience a feeling of self-importance.

Thinking positively about yourself is the first step in any self-improvement program. In becoming a new person you will begin to develop normal self-love, self-respect, self-confidence, and inner contentment. Your future will depend on this *inner self*—the way you think about yourself. You cannot expect self-hypnosis to do wonderful things for you unless you first succeed in liking yourself—the new self—the self you want to be. The achievement of this first goal will lead to the successful attainment of other equally important goals.

You Can Enjoy Better Health Through Self-Hypnosis

It is claimed that approximately 60 to 75 percent of the ills people complain about are *psychosomatic*. This would mean that the *emotional factor* plays an important role in illness. The late Dr. John Schindler, in his book *How to Live 365 Days a Year,* describes how a negative mental attitude can cause illness. If emotionally induced illness is as prevalent as it is claimed to be, then it would seem logical that the control of one's emotions, or the improvement of one's attitude, accomplished through self-hypnosis, would do much to prevent the development of psychosomatic ailments. Self-hypnosis can also help the patient suffering from physical or organic illness by making him or her less apprehensive, more tolerant to discomfort, and by increasing his or her will to live. What is self-hypnosis but the technique of influencing your own thinking to advantage— managing your emotions successfully at all times?

Many people become chronic health complainers only because their symptom-complaints represent expressions of some inner unhappiness. The person who subjects himself or herself to self-analysis, attempting to uproot the cause of his or her unhappiness (following this with auto-posthypnotic suggestions as a remedy) is less apt to become a hypochondriac.

Self-hypnosis enables you to become a better patient in time of an emergency illness. It enables you to be less fearful of an operation, to become more cooperative, and to assume an optimistic outlook during your convalescence.

Self-Hypnosis Will Help You Achieve Personality Maturity

Personality maturity implies many things. It represents balanced living, wisdom, intelligence, good moral character, kindness, a code of ethics, a healthy sense of values, the ability to get along with people, a gladness to be alive, the courage to face reality and adjust to adversities, a willingness to grow and be of service to others, and a belief in the goodness of life. It means all these things and every-thing else that reflects that which is positive, good, and acceptable to humankind.

A well-integrated personality is an asset in life. It gives you the fortitude to withstand misfortunes. People who are well adjusted are capable of doing good, of inspiring others to climb and achieve success. They console those who are in despair. We all benefit from the wisdom of those who have found the secret of maturity. But such a goal as personality maturity is not acquired overnight. It requires persistent effort. It takes stick-to-it-tiveness. It means working at self-improvement every day. It entails learning, studying, listening, work-ing, growing, and developing self-confidence through accomplish-ments—achieving one goal at a time. You must define the kind of person you want to be before you become that person. It's a matter of reminding yourself from day to day of those personality traits you want for yourself. Personality maturity, when you have it, is like money in the bank, like owning a home without a mortgage. It is mind-health, mind-power.

Successful Planning

Self-hypnosis enables you to advantageously plan and organize your time and daily activities.

Much of your happiness and success in life depends upon your ability to use your time wisely and plan intelligently. Time is acces-sible to everyone. Going to bed every night knowing that you have devoted your time to doing something constructive, learning some-thing new, improving yourself, or planning for a particular goal gives you the kind of mental satisfaction that makes day-to-day liv-ing inspiring. It gives you a *joie de vivre*—a feeling that you are mak-ing yourself useful—giving meaning to life.

Self-hypnosis is synonymous with self-discipline. It means starting the day with a healthy attitude toward the responsibilities you must face as well as knowing how you are going to organize your time and energy for that particular day. To live without plans is to sail a ship without a compass. To build, you must be guided by a set of plans. To work toward a given goal, you must have organization.

Organization means knowing what you want out of life, what you don't want, what you expect from yourself and others, how you prefer to spend your time, and what you must do to achieve your goals. It means thinking straight—positive thinking—rational thinking—thinking with a plan.

Once you have developed the ability to utilize time and energy wisely, you are ready to direct the power of self-hypnosis toward the achievement of your next goal.

Self-Hypnosis Can Improve Your Love Life

Love-happiness is an experience, a feeling within, a something you share. If you feel love in your heart, you are able to reflect it. It is easy to express something you feel. Love-happiness is essential to relationship- and marriage-happiness. Self-hypnosis can assist you in becoming a more lovable person, a person more likely to be in a loving relationship.

If you are already married or in a committed relationship, it will help you to improve your relationship to your partner. Self-discipline and self-control achieved through self-hypnotic techniques will help you and your partner to be consistent in your reactions to each other, building an atmosphere of respect, love, and trust. Self-hypnosis can help you to enjoy the physical expression of love, learn to be more responsive, more receptive, and a happy co-participant. A happy couple is one that enjoys a happy love-sex relationship. Happily committed people get more out of life. They make better friends, better parents, and better citizens. Their happiness is contagious. Improve your love life, and you will have achieved one of the important ingredients of successful living. The Italians have a saying: "A meal without wine is like a day without sunshine." We can paraphrase it by saying, Life without love is like a flower without fragrance. Love is the *élan vital* of life; love is the *raison d'être* of life—the motivation behind everything that is good in the world. Love-happiness means life-happiness. Love is something you can develop, acquire, possess. It is a feeling that you can experience by planting the seeds of love in your mind, in your thinking, in everything you do. Love is an attitude of mind that you can develop through self-hypnosis. Learn to *think love in your mind and you will feel love in your heart.*

How to Use This Book to Your Greatest Advantage

We hope that the knowledge you will gain from reading and reread-ing this book will convince you that self-hypnosis is simply a tech-nique for developing greater self-discipline and helping you achieve your goals in life. Self-hypnosis helps you to help yourself. When you finish reading the book, resolve that you have just begun your new way to successful living.

Use the contents of this book to inspire you to better yourself in every way. Practice the techniques faithfully for achieving self-mastery.

Self-hypnosis gives you *mind-power.* It gives you the ability to convert acquired knowledge into *wisdom*.

If you make this book your guide to self-improvement, you will be reaping the maximum benefit from all that you have learned.

Hypnosis: Theories, Fallacies, and Facts

We believe that for you to understand the mechanism of self-hypnosis properly and have self-hypnosis work for you successfully, it is essential that you have some knowledge of what we mean by "hypnosis." We want to briefly review some of the different theories about it, the various fallacies and facts of it, and how hypnosis and self-hypnosis are, in today's world, one of our greatest forces for good.

Everyone Has Been Hypnotized

We have all been hypnotized. Yes, you probably have, too. Have you ever caught yourself daydreaming and failed to notice what was going on around you? Perhaps you have been driving along on the freeway, listening to the radio, and missed a familiar exit. Have you ever been so engrossed in a book or a movie that you were unaware of the passing of time? These are all hypnotic-like trances.

Definition of Hypnosis

Most people have their first, and sometimes their only, experience with hypnosis through watching a stage show or other hypnosis-for-entertainment-type event. From this, they often get the impression that hypnosis is something mystical and dangerous, a form of mind control with the subject only a helpless victim. Nothing could be further from the truth.

What, then, is hypnosis? Leslie LeCron, psychologist and lecturer on hypnotism, describes hypnosis as "The uncritical acceptance of a suggestion by the patient in a trance." Andrew Salter, author of *What Is Hypnosis?* is of the opinion that hypnosis is nothing more than "a conditional reflex." Dr. A. M. Krasner, author of the hypnotherapy teaching text *The Wizard Within*, says, "Hypnosis may be defined as a process which produces relaxation, distraction of the conscious mind, heightened suggestibility and increased awareness, allowing access to the subconscious mind through the imagination. It also produces the ability to experience thoughts and images as real."

Clearly, the experience of hypnosis is difficult to define because it is a subjective matter. Nevertheless, most professionals in the field regard hypnosis as an exaggerated form of suggestibility. We choose the following definition as our best understanding of the hypnotic phenomenon: *Hypnosis may be defined as a sleeplike condition produced by the hypnotist in a subject who allows himself or herself to accept and respond to certain specific suggestions.*

Origin of the Word

The term "hypnosis" is derived from the name of the Greek god of sleep Hypnos and was coined by an English physician, Dr. James Braid, in 1843. Incidentally, we believe that it is an unfortunate term since it conveys the erroneous impression that hypnosis is the same as sleep. Actually, hypnosis as already defined means increased receptivity to suggestion. It has been discovered that suggestion has a more profound effect when the subject is in a hypnotic state.

There Are Two Kinds of Hypnosis

1. Hetero-hypnosis: the induction of the hypnotic state in a subject by someone else (the hypnotist—sometimes called the "operator").

2. Autohypnosis or self-hypnosis: the induction of the hypnotic
state by oneself.

What Is Meant by the Hypnotic State?

The hypnotic state is a condition that is somewhat similar to sleep.
Hypnosis and sleep are not the same thing. In the hypnotic state
the reflexes are present. In natural sleep reflexes are diminished or
absent.

The hypnotic state may be compared to a dreamlike state. The
person in a hypnotic state is self-absorbed as if in fantasy. The hypnotic state has also been likened to a state of absentmindedness, or
a state of dissociation of consciousness in which the subject is partially withdrawn from reality. Actually, the subject is fully aware of
what is happening and is extremely alert.

Theories of Hypnosis

There are many controversial theories regarding the exact nature of
hypnosis. Professor H. Bernheim, one of the earliest pioneers in the
field of hypnosis, who induced hypnosis over 10,000 times, attributed the entire phenomena to *suggestibility*. French neurologist Jean
Martin Charcot maintained that hypnosis was merely a manifestation
of *hysteria*. Dr. S. J. Van Pelt adhered to the theory that hypnosis is
no more than a *super-concentration of the mind*.

Sigmund Freud, on the other hand, concluded that the mechanism of hypnosis could be explained on the basis of *emotional rapport* (transference) that the subject experiences toward the hypnotist
as a parent-substitute. He believed that not all subjects were hypnotizable, that in hypnosis the subject became too dependent on the
hypnotist, and he abandoned hypnosis in favor of psychoanalysis.
However, we now know this is not true. The hypnotherapist stresses
the need for the patient to become emotionally *self-sustaining*. The
competent therapist uses the same technique of counter-transference
that the psychoanalyst uses to offset the patient's dependency.

Common Fallacies and Facts

There are many misconceptions about hypnosis. Before you are hypnotized or employ self-hypnosis you should acquire preliminary information as to what *isn't* true about hypnosis so that your fears about it may be allayed. You are more apt to respond successfully if you are prepared properly for hypnosis by knowing clearly what to anticipate. We contend that the more knowledge a person possesses about the subject, the more favorable the result.

The following represents some of the more common fallacies about hypnosis that many people believe to be true. These serious misconceptions serve only as a hindrance to successful hypnosis. They came about as a result of erroneous impressions conveyed to the public via sensational stage demonstrations, over the radio and on television. Many novels and articles have been written about hypnosis that contain inaccurate information. Here are a few examples of some mistaken ideas about hypnosis.

THE FALLACY:

A hypnotist is a person gifted with unusual Svengali-like or mysterious magic power.

THE FACT:

Hypnotists do not possess any unusual or mystical powers. A hypnotist is a person who knows that his or her subject actually hypnotizes himself or herself. The hypnotist is merely a person who knows the science and art of *effective suggestion* and teaches the subject how to bring about or self-induce the hypnotic state. Hypnotism has sometimes been called the "manipulation of the imagination."

THE FALLACY:

A person in a hypnotic state may not be easily awakened and may remain in that state for a long time.

THE FACT:

The hypnotic state is similar to becoming completely absorbed in a movie or a book. In other words, it represents a concentration of attention.

No one has ever remained indefinitely in a hypnotic state. The hypnotist or subject terminates the hypnotic state at will. It is as simple as opening one's eyes. The subject eventually awakens from what is often referred to as "hypnotic sleep." Any fear of not awakening is unwarranted. There has never been a case in which the subject did not return to the waking state.

THE FALLACY:

Hypnosis effects a cure in just one or two sessions.

THE FACT:

In many instances one or two sessions of hypnosis may enable a person to break a habit. In the majority of cases, however, it requires a number of sessions before a favorable result is obtained.

THE FALLACY:

Many people cannot be hypnotized.

THE FACT:

Ninety percent of all people can be hypnotized. You cannot hypnotize a feeble-minded person. It takes imagination and a willingness to cooperate—a willingness to accept suggestions. Reinforced sessions make the subject more hypnotizable. Children, incidentally, respond well to hypnotic techniques. The best subject is the person who has a definite reason or motivation for wanting to be hypnotized. The ability to be hypnotized successfully lies within you. It is dependent upon your ability to overcome your resistance to hypnosis. This resistance may be conscious or unconscious.

To be hypnotized you must (1) *want* to be hypnotized, (2) have confidence in the hypnotist; (3) and train your mind to *accept* suggestion. The late Dave Elman, a famous medical hypnosis teacher, included a fourth requirement—absolute freedom from fear. He said, "Remove fear—the biggest block of all—and you'll be able to hypnotize one hundred people out of a hundred."

THE FALLACY:

Under hypnosis you are apt to do anything—good or bad—you are like a slave who obeys his or her master automatically, irrespective of what you are told to do.

THE FACT:

Under hypnosis, the subject will not do anything contrary to that person's moral principles. He or she will not commit an antisocial act, has the power to select only the suggestions he or she is willing to accept, and will reject any improper suggestions.

According to Dr. Betty Scott, University of Missouri professor and clinical hypnotherapy teacher, "A hypnotized patient is never in anybody else's power. He won't go into a trance unless he wants to. He won't do anything unless he wants to. And he won't stay in a trance if he wants to come out of it."

THE FALLACY:

Hypnosis means being put to sleep and not being aware of one's surroundings.

THE FACT:

Hypnosis does not necessarily mean falling asleep. Under hypnosis, awareness is increased. If the subject does fall asleep, it is only because the person was completely relaxed and wanted to sleep; he or she will ultimately awaken refreshed.

THE FALLACY:

A person has to be put into a deep state of hypnosis before he or she can be helped.

THE FACT:

You need not be in a deep state of hypnosis to benefit from hypnosis. Many excellent results are being obtained by utilizing the beneficial suggestible state of light induction.

THE FALLACY:

Hypnosis will not help persons suffering from sexual problems.

THE FACT:

Hypnosis has proven effective in helping many persons over-come sexual problems. Many cases of impotence and frigidity as well as other sexual disorders have been reported as responding successfully to hypnotherapy.

THE FALLACY:

Persons who are easily hypnotized are weak-willed.

THE FACT:

The more intelligent and imaginative the person is, the easier it is for that person to experience hypnosis. You don't have to be "weak-minded" to be hypnotized.

THE FALLACY:

A hypnotist can induce a person to commit a crime.

THE FACT:

A hypnotist cannot induce a person to commit a crime or any illegal act.

THE FALLACY:

Being hypnotized means lapsing into a state of unconsciousness.

THE FACT:

Being hypnotized, even in a deep state, does not mean lapsing into a state of unconsciousness. Under hypnosis, you are aware of everything that is going on.

Hypnosis Versus Self-Hypnosis

As we have already explained, all hypnosis is self-hypnosis. In hypnosis the subject responds to the suggestions of the hypnotist. The subject *permits* the hypnotist to bring about a state of calmness and relaxation because the subject *desires* this mental state.

Hypnosis involves (1) motivation, (2) relaxation, and (3) suggestion.

In self-hypnosis, the relaxation is *self-induced*, followed by the hypnotic state. It is the influence of our own minds over our bodies. By inducing our own hypnotic state, we heighten our suggestibility and are then capable of influencing our body functions, of experiencing tranquility without the use of drugs. Or, we may give ourselves specific chosen suggestions in the hypnotic state (posthypnotic suggestion). The actual techniques of self-hypnosis will be discussed in Chapter 5.

The phenomena of hypnosis and self-hypnosis may even explain many of our publicized miracles of faith cures.

Self-hypnosis is, after all, really a form of *psychic healing* accomplished through the voluntary *acceptance and application of one's own suggestions.*

Self-Hypnosis in Our Daily Lives

Every one of us practices some form of self-hypnosis unknowingly. For instance, we find ourselves being irresistibly coerced, persuaded, or influenced by the suggestions of others. It would be impossible to estimate the extent or role that hypnotic influences play in our everyday thinking. Our life is constantly changing because of what we see, hear, or tell ourselves. Suggestibility is a common denominator in the psychology of human behavior. Many of the things we believe are accepted on faith. We believe them only because we *want* to believe them. Some of us, of course, are more suggestible than others.

For example, the compulsion to buy what we see and want (oniomania) operates on the principle of hypnotic influences. Something tells us we *must* have it. The picture of a delicious piece of pie on the restaurant mirror, travel pictures of Venice or Paris, or a beautiful girl modeling a swimsuit are examples of *hypnotic visual appeal*. A suggestive picture of a Florida home with palm trees and a boat tied up at a private dock, with persuasive descriptions of how easy it is to own, is another example of "let us make up your mind for you."

A manifestation of self-hypnosis is disguised in the phenomenon of being in love or falling in love. Proof of the interrelationship between hypnosis and love is evidenced in Dr. Bernard Hollander's observation:

> One of the best examples of the effect of suggestion to the extent of its becoming an obsession is that of a person who has fallen in love. It is as powerful in its mental and bodily effects as hypnotism. The man or woman who has induced this state of mind exercises a strong fascination over the subject, resulting in complete blindness to the attractions of all other persons and to the physical and mental defects of the object of adoration. Men in love sometimes change the habits of a lifetime, break with their own relations, dismiss their most faithful servants, ruin themselves financially, give up their club and smoking, and may even change their politics and religion. Simultaneously with these mental changes there are certain physical symptoms. In the presence of the object of infatuation a gentle languor pervades the frame; the respiration becomes sighing; the blood rushes to the head, caus-

ing a flushing of the countenance. Accompanying this is a great confusion of thought and language. Particularly in young persons, and when very acute there may be loss of appetite and insomnia. There is usually a disposition to violent palpitation of the heart and a sensation at times as if the heart had been displaced upward into the larynx. Persons in love become highly sensitive to each other's feelings. The slightest inattention, or a greeting less warm than usual, will cause serious agitation, worry, misery, lasting for hours or even days. They become moody and avoid society. If the neglect continues they grow pale and thin, morbid thoughts of self-destruction may arise, and sometimes homicidal impulses at the sight of a rival have been known to occur. On the other hand, a contact of the hands, and even more so of the lips or cheeks, though the action lasts but a second, may excite feelings of exaltation and happiness of an enduring character. There is no hypnotist who can produce such complex results at once as are manifest in a person who has "fallen in love."

Dr. George C. Kingsbury, author of *The Practice of Hypnotic Suggestion*, describes how Indian fakirs resort to *self-hypnosis* by fixing their eyes on a selected object and how our own American Indians in Dakota would put themselves in the hypnotic state while performing their "ghost dance" and finally fall asleep. He mentions the monks of Mount Athos who hypnotized themselves by looking steadily at their own navels.

You can prove through practice that you are capable of hypnotizing yourself. Some of us allow ourselves to relax and fall asleep reading a book or listening to soft music. Others accomplish the same effect through conscious autosuggestion and autoconditioning. Building up our own self-confidence in a way is a form of self-hypnosis.

Remember that everyone can develop into a good subject with sufficient motivation and practice.

Hypnosis and Self-Hypnosis: Forces for Good

As you know, the public has always been fascinated by the subject of hypnotism. Fortunately, people are becoming more and more educated as to the myths and facts of hypnosis. So-called "stage hypnosis" is becoming extinct, like the old-time vaudeville. Today, current magazines are reporting the wonderful things hypnosis can do. Hypnotism is proving that a power exists within each person, call it mind-power, the power of positive thinking, anything you like. The utilization of this inner force or power enables people to endure pain.

For example, hypnosis has been used successfully in helping alleviate the pain associated with terminal cancer. As early as 1954, *Life* magazine published an article to this effect entitled "The Use of Hypnosis in the Case of the Cancer Patient." Today there are literally hundreds of articles and books extolling the virtues of hypnosis for enhancing health and healing. Hypnosis and self-hypnosis can also be used to break undesirable habits, develop self-confidence, overcome fear, and accomplish many other things that will be described in subsequent chapters. Hypnosis and self-hypnosis operate on the principle that *what the mind causes, the mind can cure.* Results vary depending on the susceptibility of each individual to suggestion. Everyone can develop into a good subject with sufficient motivation and practice.

Dr. Milton V. Kline, research director for hypnosis at Long Island University, said, "The usefulness and value of hypnotism are as infinite as the capacities of the human mind of which it is a function."

As a practical force for good, hypnosis has tremendous potentialities.

Incidentally, in 1958 hypnosis was adopted by the Council on Mental Health of the American Medical Association as a viable therapeutic modality. Many physicians today are using it as an acceptable technique for the treatment of certain specific health problems. Hypnosis has also been adopted by the British Medical Association.

Self-hypnosis in particular is an excellent short-cut to self-improvement. It enables us to acquire a new way of successful thinking and living.

Self-Hypnosis Works Automatically

We like to compare autohypnosis to a laundromat machine. You put your clothes in the machine, drop the coins in the slot, and the machine does the rest while you sit comfortably in a chair reading a magazine or book.

In self-hypnosis, after you are relaxed and have freed your mind (equivalent to the machine) of your particular problem (your laundry), you then suggest to your subconscious mind (the dropping of the coins into the slot) the right attitude you need to take. You suggest to yourself the idea that after you have analyzed your problem thoroughly while in the hypnotic state, your subconscious mind will do the rest. The posthypnotic suggestions you give yourself will become *positive habit-thinking,* and the solution of your problem will automatically emerge from your subconscious mind.

Try to think of your mind as a self-healing mind. When you scratch yourself and bleed, nature forms a scab over the scratch to help stop the bleeding and close the wound as a protection against infection. This takes place automatically. We generally assist nature by wiping the wound with some antiseptic solution and applying a bandage. The mind also attempts to heal a psychological wound (the frustration or disappointment) automatically by reminding us that we can and will survive our misfortunes. But you can assist the mind and expedite the healing by giving your mind positive self-suggestions and thus letting your subconscious mind know what you want it to do for you (the dropping of the coins). The subconscious mind will do the rest *automatically.* Remember we all have *mind-power.* It can do wonders for us if we will only make greater use of it. Make it easier for yourself when you have a problem that's troubling you. Relax while your subconscious mind does the work for you.

Chapter 2

How and Why Hypnosis Works

You have heard the expression, "You can talk yourself into or out of anything" depending on what you really want to do. In the same way, you can *think* yourself into or out of anything, depending upon the kind of suggestions you give yourself. Self-suggestion is the magic key to self-improvement.

There is nothing mysterious about hypnosis. Its application is based solely on the known psychological relationship between the conscious and the subconscious minds. The subconscious, having no power to reason, accepts and acts upon any fact or suggestion given to it by the conscious mind.

Hypnosis works because all human beings are suggestible. *Suggestion is the key to hypnotism.*

Because of suggestions we subconsciously accept on a daily basis, we react automatically and often without logic. For example, Dad says to seven-year-old Johnny, "I'm afraid you'll never be good at math, son." Johnny grows up saying, "Math is just impossible for me—always has been." A woman who has a disturbing experience with a man early in life may be heard to repeat, "Isn't that just like a man? They're all alike!" A similar situation may occur when a man who was mistreated early in life by his mother or by some other female says, "You just can't trust a woman!"

Different Ways in Which We Receive Suggestions

Suggestions come to us both verbally and nonverbally. Some of the many ways we both give and receive suggestions every day are these:

DIRECTLY: A direct suggestion is any verbal statement or physical action that is to the point and given in a "command" manner.

> "Everybody stand up!"
> "Eat your food."
> "Come here."

INDIRECTLY: Indirect suggestions are primarily nonverbal motions or sound to which we often respond without being aware of doing so.

> Yawn, and you cause others to yawn.
> Smile, and you cause others to smile.
> Look upward, and you cause others to look upward.

BY INFERENCE: Inferred suggestions are basically the same as indirect suggestions in that they are subtle and often nonverbal. They differ in that they convey a message from one person to another person or group.

> Pointing a finger to suggest "Come here" . . .
> Nodding your head to indicate affirmation . . .
> Making a fist to suggest violent action . . .

FROM PRESTIGE: Prestige suggestions are those we act upon with no questions, simply because we respect and believe the authority of the source.

> Small children believe their parents.
> We believe our physicians.
> We believe our teachers.

FROM EMOTIONAL APPEALS: Emotional appeals are those responses that change a person's emotional state, thereby setting into motion any feelings or sensations that the person associates with the event.

Shouting or threats causing panic . . .

Antagonizing or "needling" causing anger . . .

Gentleness or empathy causing happiness or crying . . .

BY SOCIAL DICTATES: These are suggestions that "lead" or "appeal" to a person's desire to belong or conform. The phrases "follow the crowd" and "peer pressure" refer to socially dictated suggestions.

Fashion . . . hem lines are "up" this year.

Politics . . . that candidate stands for the worker.

Language . . . words change meaning by increased general usage and acceptance, such as "grass" and "gay."

NEGATIVE CLICHÉ SUGGESTIONS: There are literally hundreds of phrases that are repeated so often that they actually become a part of our belief systems.

You can't make it in this world unless you are rich.

It's not what you know, it's who you know.

You just can't win, no matter how hard you try.

NEGATIVE SUGGESTIONS/PHYSICAL MANIFESTATIONS: How many times have you heard or said a phrase so often that it becomes true?

He makes me sick.

My job gives me a pain in the neck.

My kids drive me crazy.

POSITIVE SUGGESTIONS: These are the suggestions you are going to learn to formulate and use for yourself to make whatever changes you desire in your life. These are the suggestions that produce self-confidence, inner strength, purpose, calmness, and peacefulness.

I am . . .

I can . . .

The Power of Your Early Conditioning

You are continually influenced by the powerful suggestions you were given in your early years, the years before you developed any true ability to reason and think logically. During those years, you accepted whatever you were told and you believed it to be true. From that age (probably five or six) you soon developed a critical faculty, that is, the ability to reason. You then could select what you believed to be true, based on your own experience or experiences of others. Thereafter, for information to reach your subconscious mind, it had to bypass that critical faculty. Look at Figure 1. You will see a depiction of this phenomenon that may make it easier to understand.

According to many of our colleagues who are child behavioral psychologists, it is during the first six years of life that you developed your strongest personality traits and behavior patterns. You learned to basically trust or distrust others. You developed a general sense of confidence or self-doubt. You established your sexual identification or gender confusion. Whatever the exact age, however, we know for a fact that our early, formative childhood years provide us with the emotional base upon which we build the rest of our lives.

One of our clients, Aaron G., spoke to us of his past. "I can still hear the unkind criticism I received from my parents when I was a child. They said I was clumsy and badly coordinated. Since I was the youngest of five children, their evaluation of me seemed to make sense. How could an eleven-year-old boy know that he was being judged by adult standards?"

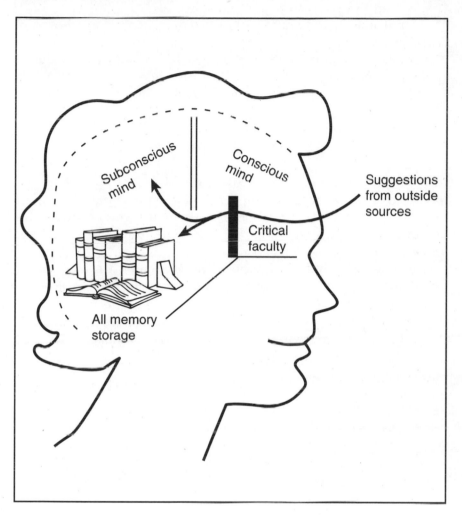

Figure 1
How suggestions bypass the critical faculty and enter the subconscious mind.

By learning self-hypnosis, Aaron taught himself to step away from the past and see himself in the present. He trained himself to play tennis, racquetball, and even the guitar. This so-called "clumsy" child had finally matured enough to stop listening to those voices from his past and to reclaim his own mind.

The Conditioned-Reflex Response

In 1904, Dr. Ivan Pavlov received the Nobel Prize for physiology and medicine for his outstanding contribution in tracing patterns of human behavior based on laboratory research with animals. In his landmark studies with dogs, Pavlov discovered how habits originate and what makes them repetitive.

The test Pavlov used was deceptively simple. He rang a bell, and then he immediately offered food to the dogs. He repeated this many times until he observed that he could ring the bell, and the dogs would salivate whether or not food was offered. Amazingly, the dogs would salivate even when they were not hungry. The bell had become a signal to their brains that food was coming, and their brains, in turn, signaled their bodies to start the digestive juices flowing, beginning with the secretion of saliva.

The parallels that can be drawn between Pavlov's dogs and human beings opened an entirely new scientific view of human behavior. In spite of the fact that human beings had superior intelligence, it was obvious that sensory signals received by the human brain set off identical reflexive behavior as that of the canine animal.

We Behave Like Trained Animals

Yes, we all do! In fact, we participate in this phenomenon daily. For example, Katy S. smokes two packs of cigarettes a day. When she drinks a cup of coffee, gets in her car, completes a meal, or performs any number of other "triggering" acts, Katy lights a cigarette. She knows that it's bad for her, but she says that she "just can't help herself." She has "quit" several times, but she returns to her habit, each time hating herself for doing so. Each time she quits, she makes a new promise that she will not return to the filthy habit. However, her return to cigarettes demonstrates the same theory as Pavlov's dogs did. Katy associates her cigarette habit with emotional satisfaction, and at the first sign of distress or discomfort, she reaches for a smoke. She also associates smoking with physical comfort, so she doesn't feel as if her meal is complete until she has her cigarette.

Like Pavlov's dogs, we respond to the "bell" in our minds, probably many times each day. Simply mention food to a habitual overeater . . . he doesn't even have to be hungry, and he will feel an urge to eat. Katy, with her cigarettes, responds to signals just as a trained animal does.

Emotion: The Most Important Element

Dr. Pavlov not only discovered and demonstrated that we become conditioned by repeated suggestions, but he also made another remarkable discovery: Suggestions are far more powerful, and acceptance of them is much faster, when emotions are involved.

Habits are often associated with emotional satisfaction. Any sign of distress causes a reach for the "pacifier" or habit. Pavlov proved that a habit (conditioned reflex as with the dogs) can be established from just a single input if strong emotion is simultaneously present. Consider the following example, which illustrates this fact for both humans and animals.

A new mailman approaches a house. The household's pet dog barks at him. The inexperienced mailman reacts foolishly by kicking at the dog. The dog becomes frightened and snaps at the mailman's heels. The conflict is immediately established. For as long as the mailman and the dog continue to react to each other with fear, the fear perpetuates the reactions, and the reactions become habitual behavior for both the man and the animal. The mailman now reacts with fear when he sees any dog, and the dog barks at every mailman.

Because of the suggestions we subconsciously accept on a daily basis, we develop a system of beliefs that cause us to react automatically and often without logic. You can easily recognize these automatic reactions, once you are aware that they exist. We see this principle demonstrated again and again in our religious and racial prejudices and in our attitudes toward specific groups of people. Do you know of anyone who automatically distrusts redheads (or blonds)? Have you ever encountered an individual who is clearly prejudiced against fat people (or thin people), tall people (or short people), and so on, and so on? Most such conditioned habit reactions have their roots in some emotional experiences of the past that are rooted in suggestion. Suggestions need not be verbalized. Silent thoughts are also "self-suggestions," influencing movement in certain directions.

Stop and consider: What are the silent suggestions you are now giving yourself? Your mind constantly turns your thoughts into bodily reactions.

Conditioned Responses You May Know Very Well

As you read the following list, notice if anything in it seems familiar to you:

> Music suggests happiness, sadness, dancing, . . .
>
> Rain suggests freshness, depression, coziness, . . .
>
> Certain people suggest joy, laughter, comfort, . . .
>
> Certain others suggest tension, sadness, anger, . . .

Some responses are so much a part of our lives that they affect our daily lives:

> Coffee and telephone conversations suggest smoking.
>
> Watching television suggests eating.
>
> A certain place or event suggests tension.

As you become aware that you are receiving suggestions almost constantly, you may notice how many negative ones you give yourself . . . several times every day. "I can't, I'm fat, I'm afraid," and so on. These suggestions have an immensely powerful influence over how you think, how you feel, and how you act, ultimately determining the level of your self-esteem and the quality of your life.

The Good News

The reason for this book is to bring you the "good news." You do not have to be limited by these conditioned responses. The same power that accepts and stores negative suggestions, the subconscious mind, is a powerful servomechanism, an uncritical, nonjudgmental servant. It accepts as literal and true any suggestion that is allowed to bypass that critical factor and enter into its computer-like system of memory banks. Positive conditioning works the same way that negative conditioning does, except *in reverse*. Patiently hammering away at a bad habit will not only eliminate it, but it will also clear the way for a new behavior that will serve you better. Remember this: *We always act and feel and perform according to what we imagine and believe to be true about ourselves and our surroundings.*

Find Out for Yourself

Close your eyes, and think of a lemon. Picture, in whatever way you can, the lemon. "See" its bright-yellow color. Feel the waxy surface of the peel and the firmness of the juicy pulp beneath. Now imagine that you are holding the lemon in one hand and a sharp paring knife in the other. When you pierce the lemon with the tip of the knife, feel the slight spray of liquid that increases as you push the knife down under the peel and into the lemon. Now, just see and feel the juice squirting out and running down your hand. Quickly, you remove the knife, raise the lemon to your mouth, and begin to suck the juice.

Now stop and observe what is happening to you. Are you salivating? Wincing? Most likely so! Is there really a lemon? Of course not. It existed only in your mind. Your mind accepted the suggestion to "see" the lemon, however, and your body acted accordingly.

Self-hypnosis will help you to use your subconscious mind's fundamental creativity: The mind will accept suggestions very quickly if the right connection is made. Acceptable suggestions are the key.

All Hypnosis Is Self-Hypnosis: The Discovery

In the early 1900s, a French pharmacist named Emile Coué made a great discovery: the power of autosuggestion, which he called "waking suggestion." Coué's famous autosuggestion formula was, "Every day, in every way, I am getting better and better." In explaining the waking suggestion formula, Coué wrote:

> We possess within us a force of incalculable power, which if we direct in a wise manner, gives us mastery of ourselves. It permits us not only to escape from physical and mental ills, but also to live in relative happiness. . . . Therefore every time you have a pain, physical or otherwise, you will go quietly to your room . . . sit down and shut your eyes, pass your hand lightly across your forehead if it is mental distress, or upon the part that hurts, if it is pain in any part of the body, and repeat the words: "It is going, it is going, it is going, etc." very rapidly, that it is impossible for a thought of contrary nature to force itself between the words. We thus actually think it is going, and as all ideas that we fix upon the mind become a reality to us, the pain, physical or mental, vanishes. And should the pain return, repeat the process 10, 20, 30, 100, 200 times if necessary, for it is better to pass the entire day saying: "It is going!" than to suffer pain and complain about it.

Keep in mind that Dr. Coué was achieving his successful results long before the theory of psychosomatic medicine became popular. Not only did he help cure various illnesses, he also converted despondent people into happy, fulfilled ones. Through his method of positive thinking, Coué transformed the lives of millions of people and started a long trend of books on using the mind for positive improvement and greater health.

He said, "When you wish to do something reasonable, or when you have a duty to perform, always think it's easy. *Make the words 'difficult,' 'impossible,' and 'I cannot' disappear from your vocabulary*. Tell yourself, 'I can, I will, I must.' "

Coué found that nothing can be accomplished until the subject's mind accepts the idea being presented. All hypnosis accomplishment occurs in the subject's mind. His great discovery was: *All hypnosis is self-hypnosis*.

The self-hypnotic trance, then, is only a planned extension of an everyday experience. The difference between everyday hypnosis and planned self-hypnosis is a stated sense of purpose. During everyday hypnotic states, you remain the same; during planned self-hypnotic sessions, remarkable improvements take place.

C h a p t e r

Boosting Your Brain Power

It is only in the last few decades that concentrated efforts have taken place to identify the source, extent, and mechanisms of the human mind and its abilities. The growing recognition and acceptance of the holistic way of life only affirms our belief that through self-hypnosis we can all enhance the capabilities of our minds.

The Miracle of the Human Body

The complexities of the human mind are frequently talked about. However, much less attention is paid to the miraculous self-preserving and regenerating characteristics of the human body. Literally trillions of reactions take place every second within each bodily cell, making the body capable of actually renewing itself. The stomach lining replaces itself every five days, the skin replaces itself every month, the liver is replaced every six weeks, and the entire skeleton is renewed every three months. Every year, more than 95 percent of the atoms in our bodies are replaced with new ones. Every second or so, we inhale one set of gases, churn it through our entire system, and inhale a different set.

Each of us has a bloodstream that contains 25 trillion red cells. It moves through approximately 60 thousand miles of blood vessels, regulating bodily temperature, and sorting and carrying properly sorted hormones, enzymes, and nutrients to precisely the right location at exactly the right time. We now know that the neurons in the nervous system are the chemical transmitters of messages from the brain to the body. Everything is controlled, from the heartbeat and motor abilities to sensory perceptions and emotional responses. Thoughts and emotions are transmitted to specialized areas of the brain, which, in turn, sorts it all out with precision.

Your Amazing Brain

For the purposes of self-hypnosis, it is not necessary to dwell on the intricacies of the physiology of the human brain. We think that it is important for you to be aware, however, of a few fascinating facts that may spark a new appreciation of yourself!

For centuries, we have searched for the answers to the mysteries that surround us. Humans have used their intelligence to project to faraway galaxies, yet the greatest of all mysteries is not in outer space. The most intriguing phenomenon is within the inner spaces of our own skulls.

Nothing that our brain has invented can come close to comparing to the brain itself. In describing the human brain, we often use the analogy of a computer in our attempt to describe how it functions. However, many interconnected, sophisticated, and advanced computers fail to match the circuitry and capacity of the brain. Its parts are connected with approximately 2 million nerve endings. Inside this approximately three-pound grayish-colored mass, 10 to 15 billion neurons store, sort, and process all of the information that becomes available to it.

The brain can be viewed as a biological computer that controls, prioritizes, and limits the use of all our other faculties. It directs, monitors, and regulates various functions of the body, acting as sort of a general coordinator. It is amazing to realize that this one organ accounts for the activity of the voluntary and involuntary systems of the body as well as consciousness, thought, perception, and creativity.

At the beginning of life, the brain is ready. It starts to record every single piece of information that it encounters. Every experience becomes permanently recorded. Every picture, sound, word, sensation, taste, and smell is recorded. These experiences become the foundation of our basic belief system. It is our basic belief system that acts as our guiding force for almost everything we do.

Left Brain, Right Brain

The physical brain consists of two halves, roughly the size of a clenched adult fist, separated by a longitudinal fissure and joined by a broad bunch of some 200 million nerve fibers called the corpus callosum. Each side is referred to as a hemisphere. Both halves appear almost identical, but we know that each half is responsible for certain functions and responsibilities. Although each hemisphere of the brain has its own specialization, and we use both hemispheres, there is substantial evidence that one or the other hemisphere tends to be dominant in each of us. Therefore, we are all predominantly "right-brained" or "left-brained."

Left Hemisphere

The left side of the brain moves and controls the right side of the body. It is the left brain that contributes to your ability to rationalize and use logic. It is strongly oriented in reality and controls language and speech. It is analytical and is good with words. It does well with observing individual things and following a sequence of linear events. When we are using our left hemisphere, our reasoning is logical and systematic, ordering facts step by step, part by part, one after another, to arrive at one and only one conclusion. For example, when we plan our day, keep to a schedule, speak, and calculate, we are using primarily this portion of the brain. Lawyers, accountants, and scientists all have occupations that require logical, sequential, and analytical reasoning. For the most part, they are considered "left-brain" people.

Right Hemisphere

The right side of the brain moves and controls the left side of the body and is nonrational. It is intuitive and expresses itself in feelings. It is involved with imagination, spatial relationships, music, art, and symbolism. It is capable of processing and combining many kinds of information at once, thus allowing it to arrive at hunches or instinctive feelings rather than at analytical conclusions. Its reasoning is parallel. We "see" things in this mode of thinking that may be imaginary. We see how things exist in space and how parts go together to make a whole. Using the right hemisphere, we understand metaphors, we dream, and we create new combinations of ideas. When we come across something too complex to describe, we make gestures to communicate more clearly. Using the right hemisphere, we are able to draw pictures of our perceptions. Artists, musicians, writers, and poets have occupations that require the synthetic or integrative processing of information. Logic and sequence play little or no part in the day-to-day jobs of these individuals. They are therefore considered to be largely "right-brain" individuals.

Two Ways of Knowing

The concept of the duality, or two-sidedness, of human nature and thought has been taught by philosophers, teachers, and scientists from many different cultures and periods. The dominant idea is that there are two distinct, yet parallel "ways of knowing," each correlating to the two sides, or hemispheres, of the brain.

These concepts are embedded in our languages and cultures, and they are present in our everyday lives. The main divisions are between thinking and feeling, intellect and intuition, objective analysis and subjective insight. Political commentators say that people generally analyze the good and bad points of an issue and then vote on their gut feelings. The history of our scientific, artistic, and technological progress is full of stories of researchers, writers, and musicians who try repeatedly to find an answer to a problem and then have a dream or "flash" in which the answer presents itself.

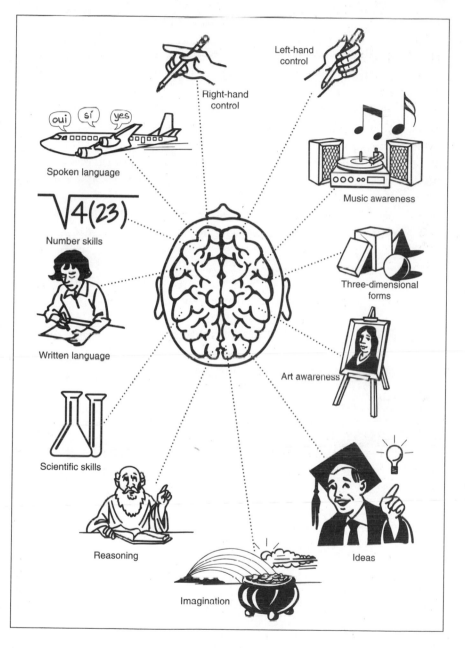

Figure 2
The Two Sides of the Brain

You may remember some of the examples mentioned earlier in the Introduction. The statement by the nineteenth-century mathematician Henri Poincaré is a vivid example of the process: "One evening, contrary to my custom, I drank black coffee and could not sleep. Ideas rose in crowds; I felt them collide until pairs interlocked, so to speak, making a stable combination. . . . It seems, in such cases, that one is present at his own unconscious work, made partially perceptible to the overexcited consciousness, yet without changing its nature. Then we vaguely comprehend what distinguishes the two mechanisms or, if you wish, the working methods of the two egos."

In another more contemporary example, consider someone saying of another person, "The words sound good, but something tells me not to trust her (or him)." Or, "I can't tell you in words exactly what it is, but there is just something about that person that I dislike (or like) very much." Such statements are intuitive observations that both sides of the brain are at work, processing the same information in two different ways.

Anthropologist Thomas Gladwin contrasted the ways that a European sailor and a native island sailor navigate small boats between tiny islands in the Pacific Ocean.

Before setting sail, the European begins with a plan that can be written in terms of directions, degrees of longitude and latitude, and estimated time of arrival at separate points on the journey. Once the plan is conceived and completed, the sailor has only to carry out each step consecutively, one after another, to be assured of arriving on time at the planned destination. The sailor uses all available tools, such as a compass, a map, and so forth, and if asked, can describe precisely how he got where he was going. The European navigator uses the left-hemisphere mode of thinking.

Conversely, the island native sailor starts his voyage by imaging the position of his destination relative to the position of the other islands. As he sails along, he constantly adjusts his direction according to his position thus far. His decisions are improvised continuously by checking relative positions of landmarks, sun, wind direction, and so on. He navigates with reference to where he started, where he is going, and the space between his destination and the point where he is at the moment. If asked how he navigates so well without instruments or a written plan, he cannot possibly put it into words. This is not because the islanders are unaccustomed to describing things in words. Rather, it is because the process is too complex and fluid to put into words. The island navigator uses the right-hemisphere mode.

Why We Don't Use Both Sides of Our Brain

Our culture is generally left-brain dominant because of our emphasis on rational-analytic thinking and verbal-expression ability. The focus of our culture has been socioeconomic rather than oriented to individual development. As we evolve further and further technologically, we are trained in our educational institutions in ways that will best serve our economically based industrial empires. We are educated in ways to help us survive in the very economic environment that created our schools in the first place.

The structure of our education has, therefore, encouraged us to use only narrow, linear thinking. We generally place less emphasis on creative processes, artistic talent, and intuitive thought. Most of our educational system is designed to cultivate the verbal, rational, on-time left hemisphere, while the right half is often neglected.

It has taken us centuries to learn about the human mind, its abilities and its potential, and we are still exploring what it can do for us. It is encouraging to note that in recent years, as we have become more knowledgeable, we have also become more aware. By learning hypnosis techniques to help ourselves gain access to the vast unused portions of our brains, we are plunging headlong into discovering our full potential.

Determining Your Own Dominant Hemisphere

Here is an enjoyable and maybe even enlightening little test you can take for yourself that may give you some insight into the way your own brain works.

Which Side of Your Brain Calls the Shots?

Nobody is totally right-brained or left-brained. But just as most people tend to be right-handed or left-handed, they also tend to use one hemispheric mode of thinking over the other. This quiz is designed to help you determine which side of the brain you favor. Once you know, you can begin exercising and building up the strength and participation of your opposite side. If you are already fairly well hemispherically integrated, you'll find it more difficult to choose between the answers in each case. To get the most out of the test, pick the answer that *most* applies to you, the one that is closest to the way you tend to think and act.

1. Think of your favorite song. Close your eyes and let it run through your head for 10 or 15 seconds. Did you focus more on:

   a. the words?
   b. the melody?

2. You're at a restaurant with a friend and he asks you for directions on how to get somewhere. Do you:

   a. draw a map?
   b. write out step-by-step instructions?

3. When you buy audio equipment—a stereo, radio, tape recorder—do you:

   a. carefully analyze all the available specifications, data, and statistics, familiarizing yourself with electronic concepts important to the understanding of the spec sheets?
   b. listen to the components in the systems in your price range and pick out one for the quality of the sound and the appearance of the equipment?

4. When you are hung up getting started on a project or working out a problem, is it because:

   a. you get bogged down in all the details, or don't know where to start?

   b. you try to do too many things at the same time and end up with your energies too spread apart, without putting your best abilities to work anywhere?

5. What kind of camera do you prefer:

   a. one that allows you to worry about the picture, and not the camera—an automatic 35 mm, or an instant-developing model?

   b. a manually controlled 35 mm SLR where you have control over the shutter speed, f-stop, flash, etc.?

6.

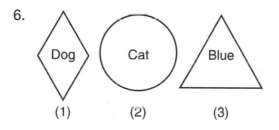

   (1)　　　(2)　　　(3)

   Does (1) match better with:

   a. (2)?

   b. (3)?

7. Are you sold on an idea:

   a. after carefully reading up on it, analyzing all the aspects step by step?

   b. if you can picture it a success, if it grabs you, or if you can get an intuitive, gut feeling that it will go?

8. Do you tend to judge a person by:

    a. what she says?

    b. her eye contact, body language, and the appearance she presents?

9. When it comes to spectator sports, are you better at:

    a. keeping score, remembering player averages, records, etc.?

    b. mapping out play strategies, anticipating where the action will be?

10.

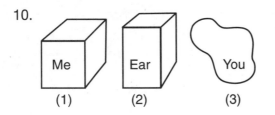

Does (1) match better with:

    a. (2)?

    b. (3)?

11. Do you work better when:

    a. you can do the specialized work that you're best at, analyzing it and making it all add up, without distractions?

    b. you can see how your work plugs into the big picture or if you're involved in interpreting patterns and viewpoints of the whole picture?

12. How do you keep your desk, the place where you work, your hobby room, or garage?

    a. It's neat and orderly. Everything has its place. If it gets too cluttered, I can't find anything.

    b. It's a mess, but I can find anything I need. If someone should come and clean it up, I'd be lost.

13. Recall what you had for dinner yesterday. Close your eyes and remember for five seconds. Did you:

    a. picture in your mind the image, the smells, and tastes of the food you ate?

    b. recite a list of the foods the dinner consisted of, using words to describe them?

14. When you buy something to read on your vacation, do you:

    a. take it along and read while others are swimming or sunning themselves?

    b. end up hardly reading it at all because you just let go, loosen up, swim, or soak up the sun?

15. When you work on a project, do you prefer to:

    a. get started right away, as soon as you have a feel for it—diving in and figuring that you can always plug in the gaps later?

    b. have all the facts so that you can analyze them carefully and plan the best sequence of steps for implementing it?

16. When you put something together—such as a game, a toy, or a new piece of equipment—do you:

    a. carefully follow the written instructions, step by step, to the letter?

    b. try to eyeball it and figure out on your own how to put it together, maybe just glancing at the instructions when you get stuck?

17. Would you rather describe an object or place by:

    a. writing a complete description?

    b. drawing a simple sketch?

18. Does your mate tend to be more:

    a. logical and analytical, a good talker?

    b. intuitive and emotional, artistic?

19.

(1) Banana   (2) Gun   (3) Peach

Does (1) match better with:

a. (2)?

b. (3)?

Scoring

Give yourself one point for each "a" answer you gave for questions 1, 3, 4, 6, 7, 8, 9, 11, 12, 14, 16, 17, and 18, plus one point for each "b" answer you gave for 2, 5, 10, 13, 15, and 19.

If you scored 10 or higher, you tend to use a left-hemisphere operating mode—an analytical, verbal, step-by-step approach. You may get hung up on details, or talk yourself into a corner.

If you scored a 9 or less, you are more right-hemisphere oriented. You look for patterns and the big picture. You tend to process information with a visual, spatial, emotional, artistic perspective or approach. Most likely you're a maverick and don't like strict schedules or structured situations that tie you down and restrict you. Your moods have a definite effect on you, and you occasionally will make decisions based on your intuition.

After you have identified your own dominant mode of thinking, you may be able to make immediate changes in your attitude and performance just by recognizing and changing negative behavior patterns. You may also choose simply to switch to opposite-hemisphere activities.

For example, if you are left-brain dominant and clearly too obsessed with intricate details, you may choose to do a right-hemisphere activity such as listening to music or perusing an art book. If it is your right brain that is holding you back, you can make a similar move in the opposite direction. If, for example, you are disorganized and out of control, writing your thoughts and plans will change your perception of yourself.

The brain hemispheres are designed to be complementary. The information flows back and forth from one hemisphere to the other through the connecting pathway mentioned earlier. Each can do the job of the other, but prefers to concentrate on its own specialized assignments. The ideal situation, of course, is to have both halves of the brain working together rather than emphasizing either mode.

You may enjoy the following exercises, which we adapted from Dr. Arnold Lazarus's fine work *In the Mind's Eye*. They are specifically designed for achieving "brain synchrony," or "mental harmony."

EXERCISE: THE BLACKBOARD

Make yourself comfortable in a place where you won't be disturbed for a few minutes. Take three deep breaths and feel your body relax. Close your eyes and imagine a blackboard in front of you. Picture yourself writing the number "1" on the board. Now, next to the "1," write the number "2." Keep adding numbers until you get to number "20." Some people can do this from beginning to end. Notice how far you can get. As you keep adding numbers, what happens? Do some of them fade away completely? Do you notice that your concentration wanders? Do the numbers remain clear, or do they become hazy? Examine your own pattern, and each time you do the exercise, try for more and more clarity. Practice the exercise for five minutes at a time.

EXERCISE: THE LIGHT BULB

As you relax with your eyes closed, imagine a dim light bulb suspended in front of you. As you continue to watch it, notice it becoming brighter and brighter until it illuminates everything around it. Then imagine it growing dimmer and dimmer, so dim that you can barely be sure it's even there. Alternate between the brightness and the dimness. Do this for about five minutes at a time.

EXERCISE: THE SEASHORE

Close your eyes as you relax and imagine that you are strolling along a quiet beach on a pleasantly warm summer day. You are barefoot, and you can feel the sand between your toes as you walk along. The sun feels good on your shoulders, and the fresh sea air is invigorating as you breathe it in. Go now, right to the water's edge, wading in now, just up to your ankles. Feel the coolness of the water. Listen as the waves are gently breaking around you. Now imagine yourself walking back to the sand. Notice how your skin feels cool as the breeze passes your moist feet and ankles. Walk back to your place in the sand where you have an umbrella set up and sit down, looking out to the ocean. See the shimmering light dancing on the water and watch the waves roll in. Allow yourself to feel the calm sensations that accompany this image. Do this exercise for five to ten minutes at a time.

While we are not aware of any controlled studies that demonstrate that these exercises do indeed result in a more balanced brain function, we are convinced that they have a beneficial effect. Why not give them a try?

The New Era of the Mind

The cultural strides of this century are incomprehensible to most of us. We've seen the harnessing and releasing of atomic energy, flights to outer space, computerization of our everyday lives and countless other technological advances. It seems, however, that even with all of our equipment and knowledge, we have somehow failed to find the most important thing of all—inner peace. Instead, we have established stress as a fact of life and unfortunately learned to rely on outside sources to give us comfort. Tranquilizers, pills, and a vari ety of cults and mystical religions have allowed us to use our minds less and outside intervention more.

For some, the 1960s and 1970s became a time to probe the mind, and a small, quiet cultural revolution began. The people involved in this "fringe" movement were looking for new ways to understand themselves and for new coping mechanisms for everyday stress. The mind was the key. People began to test the boundaries that had been previously established by society in order to understand better ways to survive and excel. It was a turbulent time of discord and discontent.

Moving into the New Millennium

The most beneficial aspect of that period, however, was the beginning of our probe inward into our own minds. The 1980s proved to be a time of growth for the study of the power of the mind. In the 1990s we have witnessed a declaration of certainty of the mind/body connection. As we prepare to leave this decade and enter a new millennium, we know that the answers we seek are not found in temporary solutions from outside sources. We are certain that the most valuable asset is within ourselves, that we can turn to ourselves for answers . . . and instead of looking for an external source for relief, we can instead probe inward to our own minds.

Chapter 4

Your Mind: Conscious and Subconscious

Self-Hypnosis Can Release Hidden Potentials Within You

Why not explore and capitalize on your hidden assets? Self-hypnosis can make you aware of your abilities and capacities. It gives you the incentive to achieve, to discover for yourself those goals that are attainable.

That self-hypnosis has been used successfully by many people for the achievement of self-mastery is evidenced in the following statement by Melvin Powers, author of numerous books on hypnosis:

> I receive mail constantly from readers of several of my other books on hypnosis telling me how they were able to achieve certain goals that they never dreamed possible. They write that they have achieved self-confidence and complete self-mastery and have been able to overcome problems that have plagued them for many years. These problems not only include strictly psychological troubles but many psychosomatic symptoms as well. Many have remarked at the ease in which they were able to achieve self-hypnosis and the results they wanted. For them it was as simple as following a do-it-yourself book.

51

Your Mind Is More Than a Brain

Your mind is a fascinating, remarkable instrument. It is a collector of information, a storer of information, and the controller of your physical and mental functions. We believe that the most important thing for you to know is that your mind is more than just your brain.

You, as a human being, are an information-processing system that is comprised of all your neural systems and every cell of your body. It is efficient and complex, and with all of our technological resources, we have never been able to create anything that comes close to comparing with it.

How Your Mind Processes Information

Your mind processes information in two distinct ways:

1. *It heeds, takes notice.* What is this? What's happening here? What shall I do about it?

2. *It acts, responds.* It sends out orders that move the body into action by sending messages to other parts of the system. These messages—chemical, electrical, and mechanical—are given on both the conscious and the subconscious level.

While we still have much to learn about the complexities of the mind, we do know a few facts. We are certain that the mind functions on two levels or in two principal areas. These areas are the conscious mind, where it is estimated that we function at the 10 percent level, and the subconscious mind, where 90 percent of our mind functions occur.

These two areas of the mind directly correlate with the two hemispheres of the brain. The conscious, "thinking" mind functions primarily in the left brain, while the "feeling" mind of the subconscious functions primarily in the right brain. This twofold nature of mind activity does not indicate two minds or even one mind operating with two divisions. It indicates, instead, an interrelated process where the conscious and subconscious or left- and right-brain activity is simultaneous.

Your Conscious and Subconscious
Minds at Work

Imagine you are spending a summer day at a large amusement park. You are eager and enthusiastic as your conscious mind takes in all of the exciting sights, sounds, and smells. You are thoroughly enjoying the wonderful and thrilling surroundings.

You notice the people. You admire the flowers. You feel the heat of the summer sun on your face and shoulders. You smell the popcorn and the many kinds of food at the concession stands. You are actively and consciously occupied with questions such as, "What ride should I try next? I wonder if that one will be too rough? What shall I eat for lunch? I wonder if the lines will be shorter in the evening?"

Meanwhile, your new, tight-fitting shoe is rubbing your foot, and your subconscious mind is absorbed in sending out the messages to your body to form a protective blister around that irritated area of your foot. Only after the blister is formed and the sensation of pain in your foot registers with your conscious mind, does your conscious mind redirect its attention to the pain: "What shall I do about this blister?" Suddenly, the focus of conscious attention is switched from the thrill of the amusement park and the lure of the attractions to a new personal priority: the painful, blistered foot.

Your Conscious Mind

"Consciousness" means awareness. When you are conscious of something, you know it, are aware of it. Your conscious mind knows of your body and your surroundings. This knowledge, this consciousness, is achieved through your sense organs. Information received this way is used to think, form judgments, and make decisions. Your conscious mind enables you to do these things by breaking down this information into small parts. It then analyzes, makes comparisons, evaluates, and forms a response to the presenting problem. You also use your conscious mind to control all voluntary bodily movements such as speaking, opening and closing your eyes, running, sitting, standing, and so on. It then takes the information you just used and stores it in the unlimited recesses of your subconscious mind. The information stored there serves as a basis for all your future actions and decisions.

THE CONSCIOUS MIND SELECTS AND DISCRIMINATES

Your conscious mind draws upon this information constantly in order to meet your day-to-day needs. It makes decisions and exercises the power of choice. It has the ability to select and discriminate between what is desirable and what is not. For example, if you begin to feel cold, your conscious mind refers to prior experiences stored in memory and obtains the different alternatives to becoming warm, such as to put on a sweater, go inside, light a fire, move around, and so forth. You then decide your choice of action.

Once you act upon that decision, the information is once again added to your subconscious memory banks. When you sleep, your conscious mind recedes and your subconscious mind takes over. However, if while you are sleeping an emergency occurs such as a fire, a sick child, or an intruder, your conscious mind takes over again, and you respond appropriately. This is possible because your senses are always functional, and they are controlled by your conscious mind.

Your Subconscious Mind

The subconscious mind is that part of your thinking that is governed by your instincts. Behind all behavior are motivations hidden in your subconscious mind.

You may have said to yourself at one time or another, "Whatever made me do that? I knew better," or "I can't understand why I used such bad judgment!"

Many of our destructive or primitive impulses arise out of our subconscious mind—fear, anger, jealousy, the impulse to hurt someone, to lie and steal. We often give free expression to them only because we have never learned how the subconscious mind operates in our daily life. Consequently, some of us have never managed to control these trouble-making impulses. Self-hypnosis makes this control possible.

WHERE IS THE SUBCONSCIOUS MIND?

Your subconscious mind consists of associated sense impressions and memories of all your past. It is composed of your brain, spinal cord, and a network of nerves that branch out through your entire body. These nerves extend from head to toe, and information about every move, every thought, and every emotion follows the route from brain to body. Every single bodily activity is thus controlled. This includes your involuntary internal organs, such as those that make up your digestive, circulatory, reproductive, and respiratory system, as well as every physical motion, even the blinking of your eyes. Your subconscious mind controls the health and function of every cell in your body. Every automatic habit and personal idiosyncrasy is controlled by your subconscious mind.

This subconscious communication goes on day and night, whether you are awake or asleep. It maintains a storage bank of memories that includes everything that ever happened to you— every experience, relationship, word spoken—everything. Not only are the memories of your every experience, good and bad, stored in your subconscious mind, but also therein are the memories of the emotions and the environment that accompanied the experience.

Your subconscious mind controls all functions of your body that are not under direct control of your conscious mind, and upon specific occasions, it actually takes over the powers of the conscious mind. For example, the subconscious mind can prevent the conscious mind from speaking, resulting in stuttering or stammering.

THE SUBCONSCIOUS IS A PROBLEM-SOLVER

"I don't know right now. Let me sleep on it." We know that the subconscious is the seat of dreams and that some dream content is the effort of your subconscious to search out solutions for improvement in your life. It does have the ability to solve problems. Many creative geniuses describe how they review a problem in consciousness before retiring, knowing that during sleep their subconscious will search out possibilities and present them with an answer.

Have you ever been stumped by a question that you just couldn't remember the answer to—only to have the answer just "come" to you at a later time when you weren't even thinking about it? Your subconscious mind held the answer all along.

There are numerous examples of creative work accomplished by individuals who moved through their activities with leisure and balance, relying solely on the knowledge that at the proper time, their subconscious minds would serve up the right answers for them. The historical documentation of great masterpieces of literature, art, and music is full of such examples of subconscious revelations.

THE SUBCONSCIOUS IS A SERVOMECHANISM

It is important for you to remember that your subconscious mind is a servomechanism. A servomechanism is a machine, so constructed that it automatically "steers" its way to a goal, a target, or an answer. Your subconscious mind has neither emotion nor opinion. It responds only from the information stored within its memory, retrieving that information very much like pulling a letter from a file cabinet. It accepts uncritically all suggestions and ideas given to it by your conscious mind, and it acts upon them with no judgment whatsoever. It cannot differentiate between what is real and what is imagined. No amount of willpower exerted by your conscious mind can override it. That is also why self-hypnosis works. In the relaxed state of self-hypnosis—which you are about to learn—you will have direct access to your subconscious mind. Look once again at Figure 1 in Chapter 2, the picture you saw when we were explaining how outside influences become part of your subconscious. This time, you may notice that the suggestions being given to your subconscious are the ones you want to give it: the ones you choose.

Your servomechanism, or computer-like subconscious mind, can be programmed, or reprogrammed, to change habits and attitudes—to literally change your life.

Your Motivation Determines Your Results

We assume that since you are reading this book, you are already motivated to give self-hypnosis a try. It is motivation that determines whether or not you get up in the morning, whether or not you exercise, whether or not you eat healthful food, and so on. Motivation is involved with every action you take.

Most people assume that their thoughts are involuntary and that they cannot help thinking what they think. This is untrue. Even the most obsessive thinking can be restrained and retrained.

The truth is that the more sincere your motivation, the more open your unconscious mind will be to the positive suggestions you will be giving it during self-hypnosis sessions. Don't forget, you cannot easily fool your subconscious mind. If your motivation is not real, if your goal is not clear, your subconscious mind is not likely to respond at all.

Increasing Your Motivation

The fact that you choose to work on a goal indicates at least some level of motivation. Sometimes when you understand why you want to attain a particular goal, you can increase your desire to an even greater level. Consider the benefits. Make a list of your reasons for wanting to accomplish your goal with self-hypnosis. For instance, if you want to increase your self-confidence at work, you might have the following reasons.

1. Make sales calls easier.

2. Be less shy at office meetings.

3. Present in front of a group with ease.

4. Meet new people more easily.

5. Accomplish more at work.

6. Be able to ask for what I want.

When you study your list, you may notice that some of your reasons seem silly or unimportant. Never mind that. No one else will see this list unless you choose to show it to them. You can benefit from writing your ideas and feelings about each reason.

Sometimes it's surprising what you discover about your motivations and reasons for wanting to change. Being more aware of your own thought processes just strengthens and increases your motivation toward your goal. Awareness also helps to dissolve resistance or blocks to motivation.

Study Your Dreams—They Can Tell You Much About Your Subconscious Self

There is an advantage in trying to recall your dreams. They will tell you much about yourself. In analyzing your dreams you are better able to appreciate those *subconscious* factors that may be disturbing your life and causing you to be unhappy. Once you learn what's causing your unhappiness, you will be more successful helping yourself with self-hypnosis.

A series of so-called "bad dreams" in which you commit anti-social acts signifies that you have destructive tendencies. It is necessary to be on guard against habitual negative thinking, particularly if it is directed against individuals. Sooner or later, bitterness against society, hatred of those around us, and unbridled sexual or criminal fantasies engender shame and self-hatred. These, in turn, cause emotional illness.

If you find yourself engaging in too many dreams of your earlier years, it probably indicates that you are retreating too much into the past. It will repay you far more to be concerned with the *present* and the *future*. The past is so much water over the dam. You cannot relive yesterday; what counts is what you do today, tomorrow, and the next tomorrow.

A dream that keeps repeating itself over the years suggests a "root-conflict." Such a conflict can color your entire personality. A person who keeps dreaming of associating with famous people or discovering the cure for insanity or cancer or of acquiring great wealth is overcompensating for a deep-seated inferiority complex.

There are people who dream constantly of falling. The repeated dream of falling may represent a temptation to go astray. It suggests yielding to your impulses. Repeated dreams in which you find yourself in a dangerous or frustrating situation suggest anxiety and fear. They may be the result of actual experiences in your past when your life was threatened either by serious illness or an accident. Soldiers often experience "battle dreams" years after the war is over. These are also referred to as "echo dreams."

To remember your dreams you must go to bed with the intention of dreaming. As you fall asleep, let your mind wander. Have a piece of paper and a pencil handy on the bedside table. If in the middle of the night or early morning you are awakened by your dreams, turn on the light and jot it down. Then go back to sleep again.

If you dream during the night, ask yourself before getting out of bed in the morning, "What did I dream about?" It is within those first five minutes of awakening that you are most apt to remember your dream. If you fail the first few times, keep on trying. We can assure you that you will finally begin to recall them. Keep this up until you have collected a series of 25 to 50 written dreams. Read them over, study them carefully, and try to evaluate them in terms of what you are about to learn concerning the interpretation of your dreams.

Treat each dream as if it were a jigsaw puzzle. When you have put together enough of these pieces, the picture will emerge. That picture may open your eyes to a new estimate of yourself—a new light on weakness in yourself that your conscious mind has been glossing over—a new light on a vague feeling of unhappiness or guilt haunting you.

How to Make Your Subconscious Mind Work for You

Your subconscious mind is equivalent to land that is valuable. Humans discovered that by drilling for oil they were able to take from the earth a priceless commodity that has been useful for many purposes. There are equivalent *treasures* to be found in your subconscious mind. It takes only a bit of mental digging or exploring plus knowledge regarding how to make your subconscious mind work for you.

If you have a problem, for instance, that's worrying you, or if you have some important decisions, go to bed with the idea firmly planted in your mind that you are going to devote a small part of your sleep time to studying and analyzing your problem, resorting to the technique of hypnotic autoanalysis, which you will learn about in Chapter 5. Will this cause you to have a sleepless night? Not necessarily. Decide beforehand that you are going to devote *only* the first half or full hour of sleep to your problem. After you have found the answer, *suggest* to yourself while still in a semi-sleep state that you are going to sleep soundly with the satisfaction that you have found the solution. You will experience a feeling of satisfaction for having made up your mind about whatever bothered you. You can utilize sleep-thinking, sleep-concentration for advantage. Your subconscious mind can give your intellect the power to triumph over your emotions. It will enable you to do wiser thinking.

The next time you are confronted with a serious problem, try sleeping on it. Give your subconscious mind a chance to analyze it, but be sure to remain hypnotically relaxed all during the time you are trying to arrive at a decision.

⇒ *A Major Frustration That Was Converted into an Asset Through Self-Hypnosis.* *

I'm firmly convinced that when something undesirable happens or I encounter a disappointment or make a mistake in a decision, I can always reap an advantage of some kind from the experience. I no longer react to frustration as I did at one time, for I know that I can profit from whatever happens, good or bad, in one way or another. Let me cite an example—something that occurred in connection with the writing of this book.

My wife and I decided to take an extensive Mediterranean cruise on the *Caronia* with our two sons, during which time I would have an opportunity to do some writing toward the first draft of this book. I had written other books on previous trips and looked forward to another work-recreation vacation.

---

*A personal experience as related by one of the co-authors.

In packing, I placed all the reference material I needed (notes, table of contents, two completed chapters, books, and case illus tration data) into a leather briefcase. The day prior to our departure, I drove to the pier to leave our luggage. The baggage master suggested that I leave everything with him but my briefcase, advising me to carry it with me aboard ship the following day. In this way there would be no chance of its getting lost, particularly after my telling him about my concern over the value, or rather, importance of its contents to me. As a result, I put it back in the trunk of my car, deciding to do as he had suggested. By now you must suspect what happened.

We were out at sea, the baggage had been brought to our stateroom. But what about the briefcase? It gave me a cold chill to think that I had forgotten to take it out of the trunk of the car the next day and that the car had been left behind at my sister's home in New Jersey for the duration of the trip.

My immediate reaction was one of irreconcilable frustration. I felt that I had ruined my trip, in a way—that I would be very unhappy not being able to spend a part of each day working on the manuscript. It soon occurred to me that if I maintained this attitude of frustration throughout the trip, letting it depress me, it would not only be unfair to my wife and sons, but I would be making matters worse by failing to enjoy myself—the primary purpose of taking any vacation. I tried to rationalize that subconsciously I must have wanted to forget the briefcase in order to have an excuse to really relax and have a good time. But as a psychiatrist, I was aware of the fact that I was merely playing games with my subconscious. Rationalizing wasn't the answer. Finally, in my sleep, the idea occurred—why can't you still work on the book? Here is a wonderful opportunity to apply self-hypnosis. Through self-hypnosis you can recall the Table of Contents, which you can use as a guide, and you will also be able to write every day as much as you desire since the source of most of your material *is* in your mind. You may have forgotten the briefcase and your notes, but you haven't left your head or your mind behind.

It would also be a further challenge to write without being able to refer to notes—I would be forced to rely on new ideas for what might be called creative or inspired writing. When I awakened in the morning, my wife remarked about my sudden change in mood and wanted me to account for my cheerful disposition. I decided to find a spot on the ship where I wouldn't be disturbed. As I sat in my deck chair, eyes closed, facing the warm sun, I induced a trance state by relaxing and suggesting quietly to myself that I would remember the Table of Contents with all the subchapter captions and that when I awakened myself from the trance state I would write down every-thing I recalled, including some of the ideas I had jotted down a month or more ago. I told myself it *would* work, it *can* work, it *has* to work—that I haven't forgotten anything—that everything was coming back to me. This was the beginning. I now had the Table of Contents. The following day as we left Madeira for Casablanca, the ocean as calm as a lake, I went back to the same deck chair. Fellow passengers concluded I was taking a brief nap. Little did they real-ize that I was going into another of my self-hypnotic sessions.

Well, there isn't much more to relate except to say that self-hypnosis had enabled me to write more than I had ever anticipated.

What was originally a frustration that threatened the recre-ational happiness of my trip was no longer a terrible misfortune, a handicap. It was instead an *asset*, like a frown that inspires a smile. I had also conquered my subconscious, which perhaps was responsible for my forgetting the briefcase in the first place. It was another instance of the power of one's mind—what self-hypnosis can do in time of a situational frustration.

What You Think About, You Become

A great philosopher once said, "The ideas and images in men's minds are the invisible powers that constantly govern them." The philosopher Herbert Spencer, said: "It is the mind that maketh good or ill, that maketh wretched or happy, rich or poor." You have heard many versions of this same, simple truth expressed many, many times. In the Old Testament, Job says, "For the thing I feared has come upon me." Our fears, attitudes, and beliefs are all imbedded deep in our subconscious minds, and they tend to become self-ful-filling prophecies.

While it is true that what you fear "will come upon you," it is also true that you can create new and positive attitudes and beliefs, and they, too, "will come upon you." You can deliberately create and develop great positive pictures and bring those into your life.

The Choice Is Yours

You are most likely bombarded daily with things other people would like for you to do. However, whether or not you say yes is up to you. You can always say no, or better, you can use the words *I prefer*. Preferring gives you not only choice, but control and mastery over events. Remember these two words when you start your program of self-hypnosis for behavioral improvement.

I *prefer* to sleep though the night and wake up refreshed.

I *prefer* to be healthy.

I *prefer* to be patient and loving.

I *prefer* to be prepared for my tests.

Exercising your preferences will make you a more assertive person and more highly regarded by everyone you meet. If you don't make your own choices, others less interested in your welfare will make the choices for you.

Words Are Important

Do you remember the childhood chant, "Sticks and stones may break my bones, but words will never hurt me?" How very untrue it was. Words can indeed hurt, and they can heal just as well. Words are powerful. Some of the most powerful words you use are those you use to describe yourself, to yourself and to others. Your choice of vocabulary can make or break your behavior patterns—and your life. Think about certain four-letter words you know that carry with them automatic stigma and hostility, no matter how casually they are used. On the other hand, consider the four-letter words love, good, life, and fine. Those words can only heal and help. Mark Twain said, "The difference between the right word and the almost right word is the difference between lightning and the lightning bug." In formulating your self-suggestions, the right choice of words can accelerate improvement and the wrong choice can retard or even prevent it.

Using Words That Work: Setting S.M.A.R.T. Goals

Dr. Tad James, author of *The Secret of Creating Your Future*, has one of the best approaches to goal-setting we have found. With his system, it is easy to choose the correct way to phrase your goals, which will become your self-hypnosis suggestions that will be received by your subconscious mind just the way you intend. Dr. James developed a system called "S.M.A.R.T. Goals," each letter of the word "smart" standing for an important goal-setting component.

"S" STANDS FOR SPECIFIC AND SIMPLE

The subconscious mind does not deal with implications or innuendo. For instance, if you ask a hypnotized person, "Can you tell me where you were born?" she will probably answer simply, "Yes." If you were to write a goal, "I would like to have more money," that goal is not specific enough. If you make one dollar more, that is "more money." State the goal the way you want it. Say, "I now make X number of dollars per month." Your subconscious processes very literally. Be specific, and keep your instructions simple.

"M" STANDS FOR MEASURABLE AND MEANINGFUL

Measurable goes hand in hand with specific. The reason for measurability is so that you know when you have attained your goal. Some people decide, "I want to be successful." So does everyone. This is not a measurable goal. Say instead, "I achieved my sales goal of X dollars this month. You do not have to set a rigid schedule, but you should indicate a reasonable time within which you expect to achieve the goal. Meaningful means it is yours, you want it, and you own it. Make sure the goal is for you, and not because you want to please someone else.

"A" Is for As if Now and All Areas of Life

When you write a goal, make it in the present tense, as if it were true this moment. Remember the literal nature of your subconscious mind. "I am well-organized," *not* "I will be organized in the near future." The power to change is in the present. All Areas of Life just means that you should strive for balance. Make sure that you are not just working, but that you take time for good relationships, exercise, and spiritual development. Make goals for all areas of your life.

"R" Is for Realistic and Responsible

Realistic means that given the events in your life that you can determine, it is possible that you can achieve the stated goal. Make the goal appealing enough to provide incentive, but not so dramatic that it seems impossible. Be careful not to set goals that are unrealistic because that almost assures you of failure. If you are just beginning to study biology, it is unlikely that you will win this year's Nobel Prize for medicine. If you weigh 250 pounds and you want to lose weight, use common sense to set your goals in attainable increments. Responsible means that your goals are good for you and good for everyone around you. It means that you are taking into account the effects of your actions on the people and places around you.

"T" Is Toward What You Want

When you write down a goal, state it in a positive way—toward what you want, not what you don't want. Be positive.

Your subconscious mind is eager to comply literally with directives it believes to be true and in your best interests. It seems to be common sense, then, that negative words have no place in self-hypnotic suggestions. The subconscious is far too literal. There are some words that you should virtually eliminate from your "hypnotic vocabulary." Such words include:

can't

never

pain

hurt

perhaps

angry

The word "try," for instance, presupposes doubt. Give your subconscious mind only the words that mean success. For instance, say, "I enjoy my children, and I am relaxed when I am with them," *not* "I don't lose my temper with my children." Your subconscious mind makes a picture of what you say, and in that case would make a picture of losing your temper since it can't make a picture of your not losing your temper.

Change can happen quickly when you word your suggestions according to the "S.M.A.R.T. Goals" rules. We've seen it happen hundreds of times in our practice. Combine those rules with the principles of self-hypnosis that we are about to teach you, and you will change your life!

Chapter 5

The 4-A's Method of Self-Hypnosis: A Step-by-Step Plan

You have learned what hypnosis is, what is meant by the "hypnotic state," and have cleared up any misconceptions you may have harbored about hypnosis. You have been told about the many things you can expect to achieve through self-hypnosis, that you can use it as a force for good. You are now ready for step-by-step instructions as to how you can relax and induce the hypnotic state so that you will respond successfully to self-given suggestions for coping with common everyday problems. You will be able to apply the technique of self-hypnosis to specific problems such as becoming more organized, getting your emotions under control, losing weight, breaking the smoking or drinking habit (or cutting down, as you prefer), overcoming laziness, learning to concentrate better, eliminating nervous tension and fatigue, becoming less moody and depressed, improving your attitude about yourself and others, getting more out of life, or anything else you want to achieve.

This chapter, incidentally, is a very important one since it is the *key* to the entire book. Therefore, we recommend that you study it carefully. Read it as many times as you find necessary. Memorize each of the steps carefully and thoroughly.

First Decide What You Want Self-Hypnosis to Do for You

It is important to go over in your own mind exactly what it is that you want self-hypnosis to do for you. Be certain that you have a clear understanding of just what you want to accomplish before starting the actual application of self-hypnosis.

We have found that the understanding of the problem at the descriptive or conscious level is a prerequisite to a deeper understanding of the problem at the subconscious or noncritical level.

Why not make a list of those personality liabilities you wish to get rid of? Ask yourself: "What are my shortcomings? What problems do I have?" You can do this by writing down questions you wish to ask yourself and making a study of your answers. The following is a sample questionnaire.

1. Do I have an inferiority complex?
2. Do I have a distorted sense of values?
3. Am I overweight?
4. Am I difficult to get along with?
5. Am I too jealous?
6. Do I smoke too much?
7. Do I want to give up smoking completely or cut down?
8. Do I manage money wisely?
9. Do I suffer from excessive shyness?
10. Do most people like me?
11. Am I a hypochondriac?
12. Do I dislike myself?
13. Do I seem to have excessive fears?
14. Am I inclined to be sarcastic?
15. What is my major personality handicap?

As we have said before, these are only sample questions. You can make the list of questions as long as you wish.

The 4-A's Method of Self-Hypnosis

The technique of self-hypnosis consists of four steps:

1. Autorelaxation
2. Autosuggestion
3. Autoanalysis
4. Autotherapy

STEP 1. AUTORELAXATION

To induce the state of hypnotic self-relaxation follow these instructions carefully:

1. Select a place or room in your home where you can be reasonably sure that you will not be distracted by the telephone or other unnecessary noises or interruptions. It will help to draw the blinds or subdue the lights. We have found from experience also that soft music often puts our patients more quickly into a state of hypnotic relaxation. You may want to experiment by selecting a type of music that is soothing and conducive to "sleeplike" relaxation.

2. Lie down on a bed or comfortable couch or a semireclining chair, placing your feet on a hassock or some other firm object serving the same purpose. Loosen all tight clothes.

3. Take three deep breaths. Breathe deeply and slowly.

4. Close your eyes.

5. Say to yourself:

I am relaxing all the muscles of my body . . . starting from my head to my feet . . . The muscles of my face and neck are relaxing . . . I'm beginning to feel free of all muscle tension . . . My arms feel limp and relaxed . . . The muscles of my thighs, legs, and feet are relaxed . . . As I breathe deeply and slowly, my entire body is completely relaxed. I feel calm and relaxed all over.

6. During this state of self-relaxation remind yourself that relaxation is a *state of mind.* It means "letting go," relief from anxiety and tension, freedom from excessive fear and worry—thinking pleasant thoughts.

7. Tell yourself also, "Self-relaxation brings me inestimable health benefits. I devote as much time and effort as I need to practice the technique of self-relaxation. I am mastering the art of self-relaxation. Each time I practice, it is easier."

The Rapid Method of Autorelaxation. After you have practiced the prescribed method of relaxing yourself each day for more than a week and you are satisfied that you are able to relax completely, you are ready to use a more rapid method of autorelaxation. This entails the use of a *key* word or phrase such as "Let Go," "Calm Yourself," "Mind Control," "Relax." It can be any word or expression. The important thing is that the word must immediately set into action the process of self-relaxation. You must decide beforehand what you are going to do as soon as you give yourself the particular word-command. It may connote closing your eyes, taking two or three deep breaths, and suggesting that all your muscles from your head to your feet are suddenly becoming limp and relaxed.

We have witnessed numerous demonstrations of persons going into a deep state of relaxation bordering on sleep in a matter of moments. We know it can be done.

Rapid relaxation can also be achieved in the waking state. You give yourself the chosen word and quickly experience a relaxed feeling throughout your body. Your mind suddenly becomes relaxed and receptive to suggestions. In the hypnotic state you suggest to yourself that hereafter, whenever you use the selected word for the specific purpose of relaxing, the relaxation will occur *instantly*. If you are walking, sitting, driving a car, you naturally are going to keep your eyes open. You tell yourself that you are completely aware of your surroundings at all times and that you are in full control of your mind, except that you are in a state of self-induced relaxation and increased receptivity to self-given suggestions. Once you have practiced this rapid method by hypnotically induced relaxation you can congratulate yourself for having achieved your first major step in self-mastery. You are ready now to make good use of your subconscious mind by giving it orders, commands, suggestions, whatever you prefer to call them. Your subconscious mind will do for you what you want it to do. By repeating and repeating a given suggestion to your subconscious mind, you will ultimately accomplish your objective, whether it is losing weight, giving up smoking, controlling your temper, or overcoming a particular fear or phobia.

STEP 2. AUTOSUGGESTION

You will recall that hypnosis and self-hypnosis work on the theory of *suggestibility*. Just as we are susceptible to being influenced by others we are also susceptible to being influenced by our own thoughts. *The voluntary acceptance of a suggestion is essential to successful self-hypnosis.*

Through persistent practice you can increase your receptivity to suggestion. A "suggestibility test" is a test to determine your ability to *accept* and be *influenced* by a suggestion, thought, or idea either self-given or given to you by another person.

Here are three suggestibility tests you can practice. For self-hypnosis, use whichever test you prefer.

1. THE EYE-CLOSURE TEST Pick out an object above eye level so that there is a slight strain on the eyes and eyelids. It can be a spot on the ceiling. Try to get your eyelids to close at the count of ten. If you experience the irresistible urge to close your eyes on or before you reach the completion of the count, you know that you are in a state of heightened suggestibility or self-hypnosis. This is the first test for determining if you have achieved self-hypnosis. Give yourself more time if you don't succeed at first. You are probably not relaxed enough.

If your eyes do not close involuntarily, close them voluntarily and follow through with the desired posthypnotic suggestions as though you were in the hypnotic state.

Here are suggestions that you can use to accomplish the eye-closure test. You don't have to memorize the exact words; just the form is important.

As I complete the count to ten, my eyelids become very heavy, watery, and tired. Even before I complete the count of ten, I may have to close my eyes. The moment I do, I shall fall into a state of self-hypnosis. I shall be fully conscious, hear everything, and be able to direct suggestions to my subconscious mind. One . . . my eyelids are becoming very heavy . . . two . . . my eyelids are becoming very watery . . . three . . . my eyelids are becoming very tired . . . four . . . I can hardly keep my eyes open . . . five . . . I am beginning to close my eyes . . . six . . . my eyelids are closing more and more . . . seven . . . I am completely relaxed and at ease . . . eight . . . it is becoming impossible for me to keep my eyelids open . . . nine . . . my eyes are closed, I am in the self-hypnotic state . . . ten . . . I can give myself whatever posthypnotic suggestions I desire.

2. THE SWALLOWING TEST   Here is another test you can use to determine if you have achieved self-hypnosis. You can give yourself this test directly after your period of relaxation or following the eye-closure test. This test is known as the swallowing test. Here are the suggestions you can use:

As I count to ten and even before I reach the count of ten, I'll have an irresistible urge to swallow one time. As soon as I swallow one time this feeling will leave me and I'll feel normal again in every respect. One . . . my lips are dry . . . two . . . my throat is becoming dry . . . three . . . I am beginning to get an urge to swallow . . . four . . . this urge is becoming stronger . . . five . . . my throat feels parched . . . six . . . the urge to swallow is becoming stronger and stronger . . . seven . . . I feel an involuntary urge to swallow . . . eight . . . this involuntary urge is becoming stronger and stronger . . . nine . . . I must swallow . . . ten . . . I have swallowed one time and am now in a self-hypnotic state in which I am very receptive to suggestions.

With this test you wait until you swallow without conscious direction. When you do, you know you have achieved a state of heightened suggestibility. The act of swallowing has been directed and controlled by your subconscious mind as ordered by your conscious mind. After the swallowing test is successfully completed you can give yourself whatever suggestions you want to.

3. **THE HAND-TINGLING TEST** This is a third test you can use for determining your receptivity to suggestions. You use the same general pattern that you did for the eye-closure test and swallowing test. Remember, these suggestions should not be memorized verbatim; just the form is important.

> As I count to ten and even before I reach the count of ten, I shall experience a tingling, light or numb feeling in my right hand. One . . . I am concentrating upon my right hand . . . as I think of it, picture it . . . completely relaxed . . . two . . . I shall feel a pleasant . . . tingling . . . sensation . . . in my hand . . . three . . . in my mind . . . I see my right hand . . . it's limp . . . and heavy . . . very relaxed . . . four . . . I am completely at ease . . . five . . . my hand is beginning to tingle . . . six . . . it's a very pleasant sensation . . . relaxed . . . tingling . . . seven . . . it is becoming stronger and stronger . . . eight . . . it is a very pleasant feeling . . . nine . . . I can feel a very pleasant, tingling feeling . . . ten . . . I am now in a state of self-hypnosis and give myself beneficial posthypnotic suggestions.

If your subconscious mind has taken over, you will find your right hand has a tingling sensation in it. You must remember after any test with body action, a direction must be given to have it return to normal. Otherwise, the light, tingling sensation could continue after the completion of hypnosis. Now you say:

> The sensation in my hand will go away, it will return to normal . . . I now have proof . . . that I have reached a state of hypnosis . . . every muscle . . . and nerve . . . in my entire body . . . is completely relaxed . . . I feel wonderfully well . . . I shall now give constructive instructions to my subconscious mind . . .

At this point, you may start giving yourself specific suggestions. These suggestions should be carefully planned in advance of the session so that you will know what to tell your subconscious mind.

How did you do with these tests? Were you amazed at your own suggestibility—or did you have just a fair degree of response to your own suggestions? No matter how much or how little success you had, remember you can do better. Yes, we mean just that—success will come. If you practice and have achieved these tests successfully, you will have experienced the first or light state of hypnosis. You can now achieve wonderful results using posthypnotic suggestions. You will begin to experience *the power of your own mind*—you will become master of your own fate. As you practice self-hypnosis and use it as a force for good, you will see that your own "mind control" can influence your habits. You will become aware of what the late Dr. S. J. Van Pelt referred to as the "Power Within."

You have learned the technique of self-relaxation and have tested yourself for suggestibility. As we have said before, the ability to do these things has always been with you—like an unused muscle. Now you are putting this power to work, possibly for the first time. You are just turning on the power switch. You are ready to give yourself suggestions for analyzing and solving some personal problem, breaking a habit, developing a better personality, or acquiring a more positive philosophy of life.

Step 3. Autoanalysis

Begin with self-relaxation. Follow this with the eye-closure procedure. Then give yourself the suggestion that you now are ready to solve your specific problem. Analyze every aspect of it. Regress as far back into the past as is necessary. Try to associate the events and circumstances in your life that led to the development of your particular problem. This kind of soul-searching comes under the category of *hypnotic self-analysis*. The term is self-explanatory. It refers to analyzing and understanding yourself while in a self-induced hypnotic state. It is valuable from the standpoint that you will become enlightened with the answers to many questions you would like to ask yourself, such questions as:

What kind of person am I?

How is my health affected by the way I think?

To what extent am I oversensitive?

Do I really want to improve?

What plans have I made for the future?

Am I inclined to blame my parents and others for my deficiencies?

What is my attitude concerning sex, love, relationships, and marriage?

You will be amazed how much you will learn about yourself. This method will enable you to realize your faults so that it will be easier for you to correct them. Take one or two questions at a time and try to think of as many possible answers as you can. When you awaken yourself from your self-hypnotic state, write down the answers in a notebook. Study carefully what you have written and try to arrive at some conclusions as to why you think and behave as you do. Remember that *self-knowledge is the key to successful self-discipline.*

Keep two separate sections in your notebook—one labeled "What I have learned about myself" and the other "What steps I have taken to improve myself." You will find that your mind will soon become conditioned to self-improvement. The good results will encourage you to continue the process. You will begin to notice that you are developing *a new set of thinking habits.*

STEP 4. AUTOTHERAPY

Self-therapy consists of conditioning your mind to positive thinking and a positive plan of action through the use of posthypnotic suggestions.

We are unable at this point to give specific instructions regarding what to tell yourself or what to do since this depends upon the specific goal you are trying to achieve or the specific problem you are attempting to solve. In other words, the details of this fourth step of self-hypnosis are actually included in the subsequent chapters of the book. For example, you will be given posthypnotic therapeutic suggestions for various habit-breaking problems such as for excessive eating, excessive smoking, excessive drinking. You will notice also that in those chapters dealing with nervous tension, depression, fears, and personality development you have access to a list of posthypnotic suggestions you can follow or which can serve as a guide to help you formulate your own autotherapeutic instructions.

By self-therapy, we infer hypnotic self-therapy. It is based on the principle of "I can—I must—I will—achieve my goal—that I have the mind-power to accept and carry out certain self-given suggestions that will enable me to overcome almost any handicap, to improve my personality, and acquire a healthier philosophy of life."

How to Achieve Self-Hypnosis in the Waking State

Self-hypnosis in the waking state can be accomplished by going through the routine of self-induced relaxation, eye closure and then opening your eyes, reminding yourself that you are still in a hypnotic state. You are now ready to give yourself audibly or mentally whatever *constructive* suggestions you wish to put into practice.

How to Rouse Yourself out of the Hypnotic State

After you have completed giving yourself posthypnotic suggestion, either in the sleeplike or waking state, you can tell yourself that at the slow count of ten, you will rouse yourself from the self-hypnotic state with a feeling of emotional *well-being*, inspired by the conviction that you are going to benefit immensely from the application of the particular suggestions you have given yourself.

Always Keep This in Mind

Incidentally, should you have any apprehension about self-hypnosis in the event of an emergency, let us reassure you that you will not lapse into a state of unconsciousness; that you will always be aware of everything that is happening at the time and will always be in control of any unexpected situation that may arise.

For example, should any unforeseen circumstance occur, let us say you smell smoke from a fire, or someone calls you for help, you would always be able to interrupt the hypnotic state automatically and immediately respond to the given emergency situation. It should be comforting to know that your instinct of self-preservation prevails at all times during self-hypnosis.

A Word of Caution

It would be unwise indeed for a sick person to attempt treatment with self-hypnosis without not knowing the nature of the illness or the cause of the symptoms. We recommend that you contact your physician first, and let him or her decide if the pain in your abdomen is caused by appendicitis or tension, or if your headache is a symptom of an organic condition, or if your cough is the result of excessive smoking, bronchitis, tuberculosis, or some other condition. We assume that no intelligent person is going to depend on a home medical adviser or any similar book for the treatment of a condition serious enough to require the services of a physician. Consequently, it would be prudent to see your doctor first. Let him or her assume the responsibility of making a correct diagnosis. After this, your doctor will also advise you if you would benefit from additional help with hypnosis. Under the supervision of your doctor, you will be able to become a more cooperative patient with self-hypnosis. You will be less afraid. You will be able to increase your tolerance quotient to pain or discomfort and manage your health complaints in a more mature manner.

Regarding Emotional Problems

Similarly, one must exercise intelligent judgment in evaluating one's own emotional problems. We know that there are minor conditions that an average person can handle by using a home remedy, such as putting iodine on a cut, applying first-aid knowledge for a minor injury, or taking aspirin for a mild headache. This also applies to certain emotional problems. For example, not every married couple experiencing domestic difficulty consults a marriage counselor. There are many individuals who suffer from an inferiority complex who do not consult a psychiatrist. Self-hypnosis is not a *cure-all*. You must use discretion and seek competent advice if you are in doubt about the nature of an emotional ailment.

An Added Advantage: The Experience of Being Hypnotized

Many physicians, psychiatrists, dentists, and psychologists who are using hypnosis and achieving successful results with their patients have not only taken courses in hypnotism, given by various teaching groups throughout the country, but have also had the personal experience of being hypnotized themselves. Only in this way were they able to appreciate and prove to themselves what hypnosis can really do. When a doctor has been taught how to induce his or her own hypnotic state, that person is better able to teach patients the technique of self-hypnosis.

We feel that the best way you can master the art of self-hypnosis is to undergo the experience of being hypnotized by a qualified practitioner. If this is not possible, the instructions in this book will be of assistance to you in learning self-hypnosis and utilizing this state for better emotional and physical health. Having attended several of these courses, we were amazed at the large number of professional people who asked to be hypnotized so they could learn the technique of self-hypnosis and how to apply it to a problem of their own.

For example, one physician volunteered as a subject before the class and was taught how she could practice self-hypnosis at home in order to successfully conquer her problem of obesity. She also planned to use hypnotic techniques in her medical practice—helping patients with their problems.

It is logical that the salesman who is convinced of the usefulness of his product is better able to convince others of the value of the same product. Perhaps this is one reason why psychiatrists are required to be psychoanalyzed themselves as a prerequisite for analyzing others. Hence, if you want to put hypnosis to the test, we suggest that you undergo the experience of being hypnotized yourself. It should convince you once and for all about the wonderful things hypnosis and autohypnosis can do for you.

How You Can Most Effectively Use This Book

You've probably heard the old story about a young man rushing down the street, violin case tucked under his arm, stopping an elderly man and frantically inquiring, "How do I get to Carnegie Hall?" The old man gazes at the anxious young man and serenely replies, *"Practice, practice, practice."*

You generally practice self-hypnosis not as an end in itself, although it is a pleasurable experience. Rather, you practice self-hypnosis as a means of effecting a change in yourself. The change may involve a habit you wish to break, a fear you hope to conquer, a chronic state you desire to overcome, or a pain you wish to diminish. You may long to be more assertive and self-confident in your own abilities. All these things—and more—are possible with self-hypnosis.

Self-hypnosis is a skill, something you learn, repeat, and repeat again until you are proficient. It is similar to throwing a ball in that while it is something you can do with ease, you can, with practice, do it with perfection and accuracy.

We strongly suggest that you first learn the skill of self-hypnosis and become comfortable with the techniques you have learned. Be patient with yourself and know that how quickly or slowly you learn has nothing to do with how effective it will be for you once you have mastered it. Change takes time and effort, so you must set aside some time every day to practice for a few minutes.

How much time you invest is not as important as the intention you bring to that time. This is an investment in yourself, one that will pay you handsome dividends for years to come.

Work on One Thing at a Time

There may be several problem areas you wish to confront, but we suggest that you deal with them one at a time, not simultaneously. There are two reasons for this:

1. The subconscious mind will handle simple, direct suggestions. Complicated, multipart instructions will not be effective.

2. As you overcome one difficulty, you will most likely notice improvements in other areas of your life. Other problems will seemingly just "disappear." The feeling of strength that comes from one success will likely "ripple" over into other aspects of your life. This "bonus" improvement often happens slightly below the level of consciousness, so you will notice it only after it begins to happen.

A World of "Shoulds" and Sabotage

Most of us can easily recognize the difference in what we *should* do and what we *actually* do. "I know I *should* study tonight." "I know I *should* lose some weight." "I know I *should* stop smoking." "I know I *should* be more patient." "I know I *should* exercise today."

Unfortunately for us, however, knowing is not doing. We procrastinate. We fail to face up to responsibility. We push unpleasant tasks into the background, waiting for "some other time," or "later," hoping that the problem or the unpleasant task will simply disappear. We fall into saying, "I just never get the breaks. I don't understand why I'm so unlucky." We repeat our behaviors and our self-deprecation so many times that they become deeply ingrained habits, at first much more obvious to others than to ourselves. By the time we are consciously aware of these patterns, we are astonished and often overwhelmed at their stronghold on our lives. We feel powerless to carry out our wishes. What sabotages us?

Remember the Power of Past Suggestions

Your current beliefs and attitudes most likely represent a composite of the beliefs and attitudes reflected by the people and things that have been in positions of influence or authority in your life. The pervasive power of the media has undoubtedly had an impact on the way you view yourself and the world around you. Consequently, you may be guilty of looking, as the song says, "in all the wrong places" for the solutions to your problems and the attainment of your desires.

How often have you said, "I would be happy if only I had _____ or if only I could _____?" How about, "If it weren't for _____, I'd have a good life," or "As soon as _____ happens, I can _____"? By placing the responsibility for your unhappiness or problems "out there" on other people or events, you are refusing to look for answers in the *only* place they can be found . . . within yourself.

Take Responsibility for Your Life

The fact is that your life is the direct result of your previous and present thoughts, desires, and emotions. Allow us to repeat: *Your life is the direct result of your previous and present thoughts, desires, and emotions.* When you begin to notice your thoughts, you will find that you automatically do a lot of negative "picturing" in your mind. These mental pictures set in motion the forces to cause those "pictures" to develop into your reality. As we discussed earlier, you largely create your world with your thoughts.

Now you have some workable tools to change your thinking and your life. The real power is right there inside you. Through self-hypnosis, your success becomes inner-directed and goal-oriented. It cannot fail. Repeatedly remind yourself: "I created my world, and only I can change my world. I may not always be responsible for what happens around me and to me, but I *am* always responsible for the way I perceive and react. From this day forward, I remember that my perceptions and reactions are always my own choice."

Making a Plan: The First Step to Success

You have lots of hidden assets. Why not explore and capitalize on them? Self-hypnosis can make you aware of your abilities and capacities, giving you the incentive to discover and achieve them.

Begin Your Planning

There's a lyric from the famous musical *South Pacific* that says, "You've got to have a dream, if you want a dream to come true."

What about yourself do you want to change? In our practice, we have observed that most concerns fall into three general categories: habits, emotions, and physical complaints. Each basic grouping includes a number of specific difficulties. For example, habits may include overeating, procrastination, smoking, nail biting, and other repetitious behavior. Emotions may include fears, phobias, sadness, depression, irritability, sexual problems, nervousness, anxiety, or shyness. Physical complaints may include allergies, pain, chronic illness, insomnia, and fatigue. Self-hypnosis can be effective with all of these . . . and more!

In addition to gaining mastery over specific physical and emotional problems, that is, eliminating the negative, it is equally important for you to remember that you can also work on enhancing talents and attributes that are already within you, or accentuating the positive. Do you want to be more loving, warm, tactful, poised, courageous, or amusing? You can through self-hypnosis. It can also help you further develop skills of your body and mind such as athletic, mechanical, mental, and creative talents.

Make a List

When you begin practicing self-hypnosis, resolve to get into the habit of making a daily list of things you want to accomplish. Know ahead of time what you are going to accomplish today, tomorrow, and the next day. To become successful at this, give yourself a posthypnotic suggestion that you will use your time intelligently— that you will devote a part of each day to this business of self-improvement, learning, developing some talent, doing something for someone else. Repeat to yourself while you are in a hypnotic trance that you achieve your accomplishments through your careful planning, your determination to succeed, and your action.

When you go to the grocery store, don't you find it much easier if you've made a list of the things you need? Your mind wants to know what you expect it to do from day to day. No great work is accomplished without first having a plan.

Get yourself a simple pocket notebook. Practice writing down your plans for the day, then for the week, for the month, for the year, and so forth. Why? Because it gives you goal direction. You must know where you are going and what you want out of life.

At the same time you are writing your goals, it can also be helpful to make a list of your reasons for each particular goal. This is a personal document for your eyes only, so be honest with yourself. Think of what you will gain when you achieve it. For example, ask yourself, "Why do I want _____?" "How will my life improve when I have _____?" For instance, if your goal is to relieve the pain in your back, you might possibly have reasons such as these:

1. Back pain alleviated.
2. Sleep better.

3. Better sex life.

4. Working day easier.

5. Quit being called a hypochondriac.

6. Take fewer pills.

7. Driving car more comfortable.

8. Resuming volleyball.

9. Be less trouble for wife (or any other).

10. No more embarrassing groans when I move wrong.

After you've made your list, take a careful look at it and arrange the reasons in order of importance. Never mind that some of the reasons seem small or silly. Remember, no one will see this list but you. You're the one it's meant to help.

Are Your Feelings Showing?

It is often beneficial when you are studying the "reasons" list to notice what your feelings and ideas about this topic really are. You may be surprised to notice that your motivations for change may be different—or more expansive—than you had originally thought. A reason that you may have *consciously* thought looked silly when you wrote it may be a very important item to your *subconscious* mind. When you bring it out "into the open" by writing it down, you might discover that it has more power than you thought.

Knowing all your reasons for working on a specific goal makes you desire it even more. That knowledge strengthens your resolve and increases your motivation. There is truth in the adage, "Knowledge is power!"

The magic formula for success at this point in your program is organized planning. If you don't believe this, try it for a month, and we promise that you will be a convert. Don't become a victim of chance. Influence fate. Control fate. How? By making plans—more plans and even more plans. Use self-hypnosis to remind yourself to make plans for each day of your life.

The Advantages of Intelligent Planning

- *Planning builds self-confidence.* You know beforehand what you are going to do each day. It enables you to develop self-discipline so essential to success.

- *Planning prevents mind-idleness.* When the brain is idle, it invites mischievous thinking and trouble. As you know, an idle mind is the devil's workshop. Keeping busy with things to be done means being happy with yourself.

- *Planning gives you direction in life.* You must know where you're going, the goals you wish to attain, and how *not* to dissipate your time. As your plans materialize, you become inspired by a sense of achievement.

- *Planning enables you to get more fun out of life.* The habit of day-to-day planning should include time for the enjoyment of life, whether it is reading an interesting book, listening to soothing music, playing golf or other sports, seeing a good movie or play or anything else that will relax your mind. To be happy, you must make plans for happier living.

Does This Sound Familiar?

Jane rises on Saturday morning, feeling wonderful and full of energy. She has all day today and all day tomorrow to do whatever she wants. Some of that time is scheduled away already with an exercise class and a church meeting, but she knows that she can still get a lot done.

She wants to clean out her closet. She has an appointment to take her car in for servicing. She has a new book she wants to begin reading, and there's a movie playing in town that she would like to see. It's also a perfect time to begin her weight-loss diet.

Jane does not know it upon arising Saturday morning, but this is how her weekend activities will unfold: Jane begins early by sorting through the things in her closet and gets sidetracked by trying to decide what to keep, what to toss, and what to donate to charity. Abandoning that task in frustration, she has a messier closet than when she began. However, she makes it to her exercise class where she runs into her friend Lisa. She hasn't seen Lisa in weeks, and they decide to have lunch together. Uh! Oh! The diet. Oh well, what harm could one little piece of chocolate cake do? After all, she did just exercise, didn't she? After lunch, Jane rushes to the service station for the overdue car service, and she is told that she needs new tires. She isn't able to make up her mind whether or not to buy them now, and she decides to wait another month or two. At her church meeting, she is urged to accept a place on one of the volunteer committees. Jane's neighbor is at the meeting and asks Jane for a ride to town, and Jane grudgingly provides it. Her mother invites her to dinner, and she will respond with an angry refusal, accusing her mother of trying to run her life. Further, her boyfriend, John, suggests going to a party instead of the movie. The book she wants to read remains unread.

Jane's weekend seems ruined before it even begins. What a tangle of decisions and disappointments! You know how the weekend turns out, don't you?

She will probably spend far too much time pondering all the choices, feeling pulled in multiple directions, and will eventually come to a dead stop, getting nothing accomplished and feeling confused, guilty, and irritated.

Typical things that Jane will be saying to herself on Sunday evening include, "I never get anything done." "I should have gone ahead and bought those tires." "I shouldn't have eaten that cake." "I don't know what to do about that committee." "I feel awful about the way I snapped at Mom." "What is wrong with me?" "Maybe if I just had more self-discipline . . . if it weren't for John . . . if only my job didn't demand so much . . . I really have to manage my money better" . . . and so on . . . and so on.

Making a Plan Makes a Difference: Autoanalysis Can Help

Jane's story is embarrassingly familiar to most of us. It is typical of what happens when we let whatever comes up at the moment dictate our lives.

If you don't take control of your life, every day will be a series of events that are acted upon by your subconscious mind. When you made your lists as described earlier, you will be well equipped to use the autoanalysis techniques described in Chapter 5. With auto-analysis, you can contact your subconscious mind and explore further how your subconscious instincts influence your everyday life. Using autoanalysis, you can develop perspective and encouragement to resolve your difficulties.

Autoanalysis will enable you to better understand your inner self. You can examine your life and your motives without judgment. Your thoughts will be more objective because they are not being clouded by the smoke screen of thought from your conscious mind. You may begin to notice how many times each day your situation is woefully like Jane's. The act of "noticing" is a giant step in the right direction. Your planning, like most other things, will become easier and easier.

When autoanalysis has helped you to sort out your problems and desires, and you've written down your goals, you're ready to begin some serious, life-changing work. Let's get started!

Chapter

The Amazing Power of Self-Hypnosis for Daily Health and Weight Control

Everyone wants good health—a sound body and a sound mind. To enjoy better body-mind health you must examine your living habits. Health experts have found that your *modus vivendi* determines your physical and mental well-being.

If you allow yourself to become a slave to habits detrimental to good health, you are going to suffer consequences. We know also that persons who are tense are more apt to indulge in health dissipations, while those who have learned to relax enjoy better health.

Self-hypnosis is a psychological weapon or technique that can change not only your way of living, it can help you develop what we like to refer to as *health-wisdom*. To achieve health-wisdom you must develop *health-intelligence*.

The important first step is to condition yourself to relax as you were taught in Chapter 5. Search out the reason why you have neglected to observe or adhere to sensible health rules. Finally, plan in your mind a course of action that will enable you to enjoy the benefits of better health.

We have outlined for you in this book detailed, simple instructions showing how you can use the 4-A's method of self-hypnosis to develop and establish good health habits and break bad ones. Remember the method:

1. Autorelaxation

2. Autosuggestion
3. Autoanalysis
4. Autotherapy

Establishing Good Health Habits with Self-Hypnosis

Remind yourself every morning upon arising that you are going to make this day a *good-health day*. Become health conscious. We're not suggesting that you worry over every ache and pain. What we mean is that you watch what you eat, how much you eat, know how many cigarettes you've smoked today, how many drinks you've had, how much sleep you're getting. This kind of daily health preoccupation has its rewards. A 15-minute self-hypnotic health session every morning will help you control the temptation to overeat, to drink to excess, to work longer hours than necessary.

Daily Health Reminders

Utilizing the technique of posthypnotic suggestion, repeat to yourself the following:

1. I devote a portion of each day to improving my health.
2. I devote a portion of each day to improving my mind.
3. I engage in some form of daily exercise.
4. I get my required rest and sleep.
5. I eat good, wholesome food in the quantity that is best for my body.
6. I observe commonsense rules about cleanliness and hygiene in my home and work environment.

7. I am mindful of my physical health.

8. I take time each day for recreational relaxation to balance my day with work and play.

9. I develop habits that help me to be a productive, self-actualizing person.

Write down these health reminders on a small card and read them aloud each morning as affirmations. In this way you will be conditioning your mind day to day to improving your health. Try it.

Self-Hypnosis: The Modern Approach to Successful Weight Control

Is dieting a struggle for you? Have you ever started a diet with great optimism, only to give up in a short time because the temptation was just too much? Do you feel deprived and frustrated when you're dieting? Do you feel you lack will power? You're not alone. The fact that the weight-loss industry is so huge is a testimonial in itself to the number of people who want to lose weight.

Why do we fail so miserably at a problem to which the solution—diet and exercise—is so clearly simple? It isn't because we aren't interested or that we don't try. Diet and health books outsell all other categories. We spend millions of dollars on weight-control programs, diet aids, diet pills, diet foods, and diet drinks. We get our jaws wired, our stomachs stapled, and our fat surgically suctioned. The concern over weight is an obsession for many of us.

You can definitely reduce to your goal-weight by using self-hypnosis. It is a scientific aid and has increasing acceptance and use by physicians. Because so many people are plagued by doubts about the highly advertised miracle diets, *self suggestion* is gaining greater recognition as a more desirable means of developing new lifelong sensible eating habits and maintaining weight control.

Overeating Is a Form of "Psychic Suicide"

Overeating in some respects can be regarded as a vicarious form of suicide. We frequently encounter overweight individuals who have a fatal "eat-and-be-merry-for-tomorrow-we-die" philosophy of life. They have somehow managed to become indifferent to the health complications resulting from too much food.

It is an established fact that obesity shortens your life span. It is a serious and unnecessary health hazard. Insurance companies and statisticians, for example, report that a person who is overweight and is past middle life is more apt to succumb to premature death from such conditions as coronary thrombosis, diabetes, and arteriosclerosis than a person in the same age group whose weight is average or below average. They also point out that a person with a 20 percent increase in weight over normal and who is 45 years of age has increased his or her mortality risk 30 percent; an increase in weight of 40 percent over normal in the same person increases the comparative mortality risk 80 percent.

Yet despite this risk to life, there are millions of Americans who are doing nothing about their overweight problem. They continue to "dig their graves with their teeth," so to speak.

The Power of Suggestion—Again!

In Chapter 2 we taught you about the awesome power of suggestions. Not in any other realm of our lives is suggestion so powerful as it is in the area of appearance and weight. You can go to any magazine rack in the country, and on the cover of most of the women's, men's, and health-type publications will be a headline about a new weight-loss diet or method. Infomercials for miracle-producing exercise machines proliferate on the television. *These are all suggestions.* Some are subtle, some are not so subtle. Whatever their degree of discretion, they all say the same thing. "Thinner is better." "Trimmer is prettier." "Muscles make you more handsome."

Most of us also grew up with well-meaning family members and friends giving us suggestions and helping us form our attitudes about food. Some of the following may sound familiar. "You worked hard today. You deserve a treat." "Here, eat this. You'll feel better." "Aren't you hungry right now?" "You must have a piece of this pie . . . I baked it just for you." "If you are really good today, you can have an ice-cream sundae." "Eat everything on your plate, or you'll get no dessert."

Every time a suggestion is repeated, it is reinforced, and becomes more and more powerful.

Our patient Tom told us, "When I was a kid, my family thought it was so cute the way I would eat everything. I would even clean up the leftovers on other people's plates. When I got older, they started to ridicule me. Being a fat teenager was one of the saddest times of my life."

Through self-hypnosis, Tom conquered his habit of overeating. The days of being humiliated and hating himself are behind him. Instead, he greets each day with vigor and enthusiasm. This story can be yours.

Lose the "Diet" Mentality

Since we know that "diets" don't work, let's just forget about the concept of being on a diet. When you're "on" a diet, there's a subtle suggestion of someday being "off" the diet. Your goal must encompass more than just losing weight. Think instead of the longer-lasting, far-reaching goal of a healthy, happy, productive life.

The Emotional Issue of Weight

It is a well-established fact that there is a relationship between emotions and food. We know from observing hundreds of our patients over many years that people who have a difficult time losing weight and keeping it off are likely to have developed habits of eating that are based more on emotions than on hunger.

The wife of a patient reported to us that whenever her extremely overweight husband was emotionally upset, he would walk out of the house and go to the nearest ice-cream parlor. There he would proceed to eat as much ice cream as he could. Afterwards, in addition to feeling physically ill, he would be so full of self-loathing that he could hardly function. He used food as an escape. By working on his emotional problems first and recognizing that he was using food for nurture instead of nutrition, he was able to begin his successful self-hypnosis program.

Calories Do *Count. . . . However . . .*

It is a fact. If you consume too many calories, you gain weight. If you decrease your caloric intake, you lose weight. If you stop exercising, you gain weight. If you exercise more, you lose weight. That's no news to you. You've known that for years. All those special diets and exercising miracles may also work. However, only when you understand that there is an emotional component in weight control can you expect satisfying and permanent results. Dieting is *mental.*

A Nine-Step Program for Weight Reduction

STEP 1:   Devote the initial session of self-hypnosis to making a *definite decision* about your weight problem. Get yourself completely relaxed, induce the hypnotic state, and begin by admitting to yourself that you *have* a problem (assuming that you are overweight) and that you need to do something about it, beginning *right now.*

Note: There *never* must be any doubt in your mind that you *can* lose weight.

The right mental attitude (an enthusiastic determination to achieve your goal) gets you off to a good start. Remember that mind-power is based on the will to succeed.

STEP 2:   Give yourself the posthypnotic suggestion that the best way to start is to schedule a complete physical examination by your physician. Make sure that you have a clean bill of health to begin your weight-loss program.

STEP 3:   Explore your reasons for wanting to reduce—all the facts you know to be true about the perils of being overweight.

STEP 4:   Establish your *motivation* for wanting to lose weight. How will your life improve when you lose weight? Repeat to yourself over and over all the reasons why you would like to reduce.

STEP 5:   Analyze your eating habits. Ask yourself: "How often do I eat? What foods do I eat? How much do I eat? Where are most of my excess calories coming from?"

STEP 6:   Determine the reason you overeat, eat the wrong foods, or indulge in between-meal nibbling. This entails more self-analysis—more self-questioning: "Do I eat to excess because of frustration of some kind?" "Am I unhappy?" "Am I starved for love?" "Is it emotional hunger?" "Am I trying to make food a substitute for something else?" "Am I regressing to childhood when I once ate too much cake, ice cream, and candy?" "Am I overweight because of repressed unhappiness?" "Is my obesity caused by feelings of hostility?"

STEP 7:   To diet successfully, educate yourself about food. Know all about calories and food values. Know at the end of each day if you exceeded your caloric-intake need for that particular day. With the aid of self-hypnosis, you can condition your mind through autorelaxation and posthypnotic suggestion that inappropriate eating is a habit, and that habits can be controlled or broken by the power of self-hypnotic suggestion.

STEP 8:   Plan what you will eat every day. Weigh yourself daily. Keep your weight-reducing goal constantly in mind. Keep a weekly progress record. See your weight curve come down. Reward yourself with new clothing, a movie, a new CD, or a massage. Take pride in your appearance. You'll find that when your friends comment on how well you look, how different you look, your ego will be where it should be. You'll have no reason to feel inferior or self conscious because of excess fat.

STEP 9:   Repeat daily that you are becoming your ideal weight, that you have now developed new eating habits, sensible ones, and that you are no longer susceptible to temptation, *that your mind is*

*in command at all times—that you can still enjoy good food and eat
well while maintaining your weight.*

⇒ *This Nine-Step Weight-Reduction Program Works.*   Dr. X is
a practicing physician in his middle fifties, about five feet, nine inches tall, happily married, and the proud father of two fine boys. He
loves good food, foreign wines, and exotic desserts. When he
weighed himself upon returning from a restful vacation, however, he
was surprised to discover that he weighed 210 pounds. Being a
physician, he needed no one to tell him that for his age and height
this was a potentially dangerous weight. About ten years ago he had
what he himself diagnosed as a coronary attack. The electrocardio-
gram findings were suspicious. Despite warnings from a colleague
who was a heart specialist, he continued to eat more than his body
required. He made unsuccessful efforts to lose weight. Worried that
he might suffer another heart attack, he decided to stop at the Mayo
Clinic while on vacation and get a thorough physical checkup. He
was given good news and bad news. The good news was that his
heart was in good condition and there was nothing in his electrocar-
diogram to indicate any coronary condition. The bad news was that
he had a diaphragmatic hernia, or "hiatal hernia," and a slightly ele-
vated blood-sugar level. He was instructed to go on a 1000-calorie
per-day bland diet and lose 37 pounds. Dr. X. was told that if he did-
n't lose weight, he was inviting complications that would make him
a bad surgical risk in the event he had to undergo an emergency
operation for a strangulated or ulcerated hernia. All this frightened
him, to be sure, but not enough for him to adhere to his diet. He had
read a lot about the wonderful results that people were getting with
hypnosis, especially in weight loss. He was self-conscious about his
excessive weight because although he had helped his patients to
reduce, he had not followed his own advice. Dr. X. made up his
mind to try hypnosis. Hypnosis had always fascinated him. He read
many books on the subject, and as a consequence he proved to be
a good hypnotic subject. He was cooperative and receptive. He mastered the technique of self-hypnosis and gave himself a daily 15-
minute session. He practiced self-hypnosis in the waking state. He
could induce the hypnotic state in a matter of minutes and bring him-

self out in an equal amount of time. Because of this ability to allow his subconscious to influence his conscious mind, he was able to say "no" whenever someone tried to tempt him by offering him a second helping or a dessert that was not included in his diet.

If you were to see him today, minus 37 pounds, you would never believe he was the same person. He committed to memory the nine-step weight-reduction program, and carried out each step. He started with Step 1 by admitting he had a weight problem, that he would always be prone to becoming obese, and that he was going to do something about it, not tomorrow but today. He was pleased that he had had a thorough physical checkup (Step 2) and that he knew how he stood as far as the findings were concerned.

As for Step 3, he was already aware of the hazards of obesity. After all, he was a physician and had treated many patients who had developed health complications because of being overweight.

He had the *motivation* that is needed to lose weight (Step 4). Loving life as he does, he did not want to deliberately curtail his life span.

In analyzing his eating habits (Steps 5 and 6), he discovered that his compulsive eating was associated with tension, which he especially built up when he saw too many patients. Although he boasted that he never allowed his patients to upset him, subconsciously he experienced inner tension. He tried to counteract the strain of a large practice with pleasurable foods. It was the habit of late snacks, the second martini, and the occasional ice-cream sundae that did the damage.

He became a diet and nutrition expert (Step 7) and learned to avoid foods he shouldn't have.

In Step 8, he agreed that he would have to weigh himself every day—that it is easier to lose that extra one pound than to battle taking off 10 pounds or 37 as he did originally. He claimed he could never adequately describe how wonderful it felt to look good in a smaller-size suit and how much more energy he feels after shedding all the excess baggage.

Some people confess that they became depressed after losing quite a bit of weight. Our physician friend experienced the opposite reaction. He developed a feeling of well-being. He took greater pride in his appearance and rewarded himself with an entire new wardrobe. His wife and children frequently comment on how well he looks.

We're sure you'll agree with us that he deserves to be congratulated. It's not what hypnosis did for him. It's what he accomplished through autohypnosis—what he did himself for himself. He realized the wisdom of repeating to himself during his sessions of self-hypnosis "Physician—Heal Thyself."

What Losing Weight the Self-Hypnosis Way Will Do for You

1. It will improve your appearance.
2. It will prolong your life.
3. It will keep you from developing complications associated with obesity, such as hardening of the arteries, coronary disease, diabetes, and so forth.
4. It will change your personality by giving you greater self-confidence, a sense of pride, a feeling of accomplishment.
5. It will increase your energy.
6. It will decrease your stress.
7. It will give you the inspiration to conquer other challenging problems.
8. It will diminish chronic health complaints.
9. It will increase your power to cope with daily life.
10. It will enable you to help and encourage others to lose weight by your becoming an example of what you've been able to achieve through your own efforts.

➡ *How Mrs. Winston Used Self-Hypnosis to Conquer Her Weight Problem.*   Mrs. Winston had read our article on self-hypnosis, which had been published in *The American Weekly,* describing how one can break undesirable habits such as overeating, nail biting, and compulsive drinking. Having tried everything without success, she made up her mind that she was going to subject herself to be hypnotized and to learn about self-hypnotic methods of weight-control.

We asked her to write for us the story of her struggle to lose weight.

My problem was one of overweight. All the members of my family have had a tendency to accumulate excess fat from the age of approximately 28 until they developed some illness, which forced them to diet. I have always been healthy so I did not have the same incentive to lose weight as my sisters and brother had, but other factors contributed to my desire to lose weight. I was uncomfortable both mentally and physically, my clothes were too tight, and I disliked having to buy larger and larger dresses most of which were frumpy looking or expensive. My feet, which, strangely enough, remained the same size, protested the increasing burden I placed upon them by reminding me constantly, through pain, of the load I expected them to support. It was awkward for me to get in or out of cars and once I was in, it was almost impossible for me to shift my position.

Although I tried, sporadically, to lose weight by dieting, I was not able to shed many pounds, so finally I asked the advice of a doctor. He told me my difficulty was caused by a malfunctioning of my thyroid gland. He prescribed thyroid to speed up my metabolism and diet pills to help me curb my appetite. In addition, he put me on a low-calorie diet. When I followed this program, I would lose weight, only to regain it whenever I stopped taking the medicine.

In 30 years, I went to six doctors in various parts of the country, and they all concurred in the diagnosis and the treatment for my condition. The main trouble was that my system would build up a tolerance for the medicine, and then the doses had to be increased. I kept cutting down on the types of food I ate—fats, sugars, starches—but I found that as I approached a weight that would be right for me to maintain, it became ever more difficult to achieve my goal, and I had to cut down more and more on my intake. Luckily, the medicine had only one harmful effect that was apparent: My jaws ached from being clenched all the time.

During the 30 years of my various up-and-down cycles, I went up to 196 pounds, down to 160, up to 190, down to 180, up to 186, down to 170, up to 197, down to 160, up to 231, down to 173, and up to 219.

Last August, I had a complete physical examination by an excellent doctor and friend who told me my metabolism was a little high. That meant that no longer could I rely on any medicine to help me lose weight. I felt that now for reasons of health, it was necessary to get down to normal size because the amount of sugar in my blood was slightly above normal. Here I was at 215 pounds and faced with the problem of losing 60 of them without the medicine to assist me.

I had explored various short-cut and fad methods for reducing, but after an initial rapid loss, up would go my weight and appetite. It seemed to me that every friend I had and all the advertisers were in league against me. Even my doctor friend, who had spent much of his time trying to get my weight down, would load my plate with succulent food on holidays. My friends were actually trying to kill me with sweetness by tempting me with delicious meals, candy, alcoholic drinks, and huge pieces of calorie-laden cake. Most social activities include feasting of some kind. It's hard to imagine ball games, circuses, or carnivals without hot dogs, popcorn, ice cream, peanuts, and other food enemies.

I had heard about the use of hypnosis as a means of strengthening will power. I considered consulting a psychologist to solicit his or her aid in assisting me to follow a regime of semistarvation, which I expected to be quite rugged. The main reason I had delayed in seeking such help was because I wasn't sure whom I should consult.

In the meantime, my weight was gradually increasing, and when it reached 219 pounds, I finally phoned and made an appointment with Mr. Joseph R. Berger, the co-author of the article on hypnosis that I had read.

My first visit to see him took place about the middle of February, and the time was spent in getting acquainted. He asked about my health, and when I assured him that a recent physical examination by a reputable doctor had proved me to be reasonably healthy for my age and weight, he decided to help me, but it wasn't until the next visit, on February 22, that he began hypnosis.

I had always assumed that a hypnotist put a patient in a deep trance, during which he made strong suggestions, and that these suggestions could be followed without much effort. He explained that the subject is not only conscious at all times, but that she must cooperate fully with the hypnotherapist if she expects to get favorable results; that she must put complete faith in the method employed and in her ability to surmount her problems; that she must have confidence in the hypnotist; and that she must control her natural tendency to "resist."

At first the going was rough. I cut down on the number of calories I consumed daily, but I was expecting a miracle, which didn't take place. He told me to follow my doctor's advice in selecting a diet and in everything else that concerned physical health. Although I did not lose much weight at first, I persisted in my efforts. I had decided that I would continue for about six months even if I didn't lose a pound. Meanwhile, he was probing the inner recesses of my subconscious in order to determine the cause of my obesity. He used the positive method of persuasion. He emphasized the pleasant aspects of having a slender figure. He discovered that my main motivation was comfort, freedom from pain, and ease of movement.

In my effort to get my weight down, I turned at last to self-analysis in order to discover the reason for my resistance. After a while I began to understand that the cause of my block originated in my childhood.

My parents were strict disciplinarians. All of us, my brothers and sisters as well, were never cajoled into doing things. We were expected to follow certain prescribed rules of acceptable behavior. Any transgression from these rules brought swift and certain punishment. As a child, my reaction to the harshness of this treatment took the form of overeating. And once this pattern was established it continued into my adult life.

Just before each meal I practice placing myself in a hypnotic state according to the way I have been taught. During these pre-meal three- to five-minute sessions, I remind myself of the reasons why I want to lose weight, the harmful consequences of being fat, and the confidence I have developed of being able to eat sensibly, choosing carefully what I eat, and controlling the amount of food I eat. My self-hypnotic sessions might be compared to the practice of saying grace before each meal. It requires so little effort and the results have been very encouraging.

I am pleased to say that I have been losing weight steadily and to date have lost 50 pounds. My doctor is pleased with what I have achieved. He found me in better health than I was before my latest reducing venture. In fact, my health is perfect. My feet can endure more than they could last year, and I find it much easier to move about in small spaces. I am much more interested in wearing jewelry, shopping for new clothes, trying new hairstyles, and in experimenting with makeup.

I have complete faith in self-hypnosis. I have tried it, and it works. I have given away all my larger clothes. During the former up-and-down cycles, I used to store the large dresses to have them handy for the "up half" of the round. But now, as soon as I discover that I am putting on weight, I resort to a few self-hypnotic sessions and I quickly come down to my desired weight.

⟹ *A Case of Emotional Hunger.*   One of our patients, Lillian, related that she would sometimes drink a bottle of maple syrup whenever she was depressed and unhappy. She claimed that she was unable to control her craving for sweets. During her depressed spells, she would consume a quart of ice cream or eat a box of chocolates.

As you might surmise, she was 30 pounds overweight. This mania for sweets was a symptom of her *emotional immaturity*. She had a pretty face and was very narcissistic despite her dislike of her obesity. She admitted that during childhood and adolescence she had never been taught self-discipline, was allowed to eat everything and anything, and was given whatever she requested.

As an adult, Lillian had never been able to establish a normal relationship with the opposite sex. She feared marriage and at the same time spoke of being "starved for affection." She craved the same attention from strangers that she had received from her parents. Whenever she met with rejection she withdrew into herself and overindulged in an orgy of pastries and sweets to gratify what might be diagnosed as "emotional hunger."

We taught her techniques of self-hypnosis as outlined in this book. She learned to apply the insight she gained and happily discovered that she could control her craving for sweets. Self-hypnosis also helped her to prevent tension, depression, and moodiness, which had acted as opposing factors in her battle to lose weight.

You Have the Power

You have learned a lot in this chapter. You may feel that since you have failed so often in the past when you attempted to diet, you are doomed to failure again. That is absolutely wrong. Just think: You have had the willpower and determination to try hundreds of diets, even in the face of continued defeat. In spite of all that, you haven't given up. It is that same willpower and determination that has made you want to try self-hypnosis. And it is precisely that determination that will assure your success. Congratulate yourself, and move on to your ideal weight!

Self-Hypnosis, Smoking, Alcohol, and Drugs

Many heavy smokers find it difficult to stop smoking only because they have never taken the time to study everything they need to know about the smoking habit. Some feel that smoking is relaxing. Others think that a person who abruptly gives up smoking will become irritable and difficult to live with, gain weight, or even suffer a nervous breakdown. To this group also belong those who believe that they "just can't give up smoking"—that they "don't have the kind of willpower it takes."

Facts About Smoking: The Bad News

If you harbor any misconceptions about tobacco and its effect on your health, it is naturally going to be more difficult for you to stop smoking. There is no longer denial by anyone with a modicum of intelligence that cigarettes are directly responsible for lung cancer. We also know with scientific certainty that emphysema and other breathing disorders are common ailments among smokers. Just in case you need a few more negative facts about smoking, however, review the following:

1. Cigarettes contain dangerous, poisonous chemicals and hazardous compounds. In addition to the poisonous nicotine, you

are also inhaling benzene, sulfurs, nitrites, ammonia, hydrogen cyanide, vinyl chloride, formaldehyde, cadmium, nitrosamines, volatile alcohols, and urethane, just to name a few.

2. The dangers of cigarettes reach far beyond the lungs in your body. Once these poisons are inhaled, they are taken into your blood where they accelerate the formation of arterial deposits associated with hardening of the arteries.

3. In addition to your respiratory system and circulatory system, smoking is frequently associated with ulcers and gastrointestinal problems. Add your digestive system to the list. These are by no means all of the health risks. If you want a comprehensive and complete picture of the negative aspects of smoking, contact your area office of the American Cancer Association or the American Lung Association. They have a wealth of such information.

4. Tobacco smells terrible. It clings to your clothes, your hair, and your body. A smoker's breath is almost always unpleasant. It discolors your teeth.

5. Smoking is messy. Ashes everywhere, ugly cigarette butts littering ashtrays in your home and car, and little burn holes in most of your clothing are all more negative facts of your life as a smoker.

Facts About Not Smoking: The Good News

1. You can quit smoking with self-hypnosis. Smoking is an acquired habit, and habits can be changed. We have seen thousands of smokers become nonsmokers.

2. Stopping smoking is not a matter of willpower. It's more of a matter of deconditioning and of developing insight into the reasons you smoke.

3. Once you've made the decision not to smoke, you enlist the cooperation of your powerful subconscious mind.

4. Even if you have tried to quit and failed before, if your decision is firm, you will succeed this time. Just consider your previous attempts as preparatory to this time.

5. If you want to quit, but you think you would feel more comfortable with a reason that is based on something besides negative facts and foreboding threats, you're in the right place. What you need to succeed is simply a plan and a method for converting your desire into positive action.

What about all the damage you've done to your body? More good news. The negative consequences of smoking are halted and sometimes even reversed when you stop smoking. In time, even your lungs will regenerate themselves to an appropriate level of health for your age. *It is never too late to quit.* Now is the perfect time.

Smoking: It's Just a Habit

Have you ever thought about how many times you have lighted a cigarette? If you're smoking a pack of cigarettes a day, that's 20 times a day. Multiply that by 365 for the number of times a year, and, well, you get the idea. The next time you light one, notice when and where you do it. Is it upon awakening? Having a cup of coffee? Getting ready for work? After a meal? Riding in your car? You probably have a predictable pattern for your smoking habit. You have repeated these actions so often that they have been accepted by your subconscious mind as how things are "supposed to be" at those particular moments. When you deviate from your pattern, your subconscious mind senses the difference, and it causes a tension to begin building in your body so that you will take notice and "fix" it with a cigarette.

If you are like most smokers, the cigarette smoking represents a mental or physical break from your daily routine. The "break" has been repeated so many hundreds of times that it has become an important diversion recognized by your subconscious as necessary for your comfort and pleasure. Just remember that you have not always been a smoker. You started smoking by choice, and you can quit by choice.

Why Did You Start?

Think about when you first started smoking. Can you remember what it was about the cigarette that was attractive to you? Did you think it made you appear "cool?" More mature? Was there pressure from your peers? Did your parents forbid it? Were they smokers themselves?

You probably began smoking in adolescence. Studies done by the United States Surgeon General's office say that over 85 percent of all smokers begin before they are 20 years old, and 60 percent of those began prior to age 16. You know that during your adolescent years, you made decisions based on inadequate or just wrong information. When you are making your plan to stop smoking, be sure to remind yourself that you have the right to revisit that earlier decision and reverse it if you wish.

Suggestions to Follow if You
Want to Stop Smoking

Many of the suggestions mentioned in the nine steps for weight control also apply to breaking the tobacco habit.

Here are some specific instructions to follow if you wish to stop smoking:

1. During one of your sessions of self-induced relaxation, tell yourself that you have made a *final* decision to stop smoking and that you are going to start *now*, not tomorrow or the next day, and that you aren't going to allow any exceptions.

2. Repeat to yourself daily *why* you wish to stop smoking entirely. *The motivational factor is very important in any habit breaking.*

3. Convince yourself: "Becoming a nonsmoker can only improve my health."

4. Give yourself the posthypnotic suggestion that you no longer need to purchase cigarettes and that you always refuse the offer of a cigarette from another person.

5. Become preoccupied with the thought that the longer you abstain, the easier it will be to give up smoking permanently.

6. Suggest to yourself that you feel proud of yourself—you experience a feeling of well-being and that the conquest of this habit makes it easy for you to improve your life in many areas.

7. Keep a record of your progress. During each session of self-hypnosis remind yourself that you have abstained successfully so many days, weeks, or months, as the case may be. This will tend to encourage you and give you the incentive to continue with your successful self-discipline.

8. Tell yourself over and over that no habit is stronger than the power of your mind—the same mind that caused the habit to take hold in the first place. Accept it as a challenge.

9. Never get discouraged or become impatient. Habit breaking entails patience, perseverance, and determination.

10. If you must find a substitute for smoking, try chewing gum or sucking on a Lifesaver or mint. Acquire new and less harmful habits.

11. Suggest away the *desire* to smoke and the habit itself will vanish. Tell yourself, "I really don't enjoy smoking. It's just a habit."

12. When you change your way of thinking and living through self-hypnosis, you will find it easier to change your habits as well.

13. As a nonsmoker, prove to yourself that you get more fun out of life than the habitual smoker.

14. Make a list of all the advantages of not smoking and refer to it as frequently as you need to.

➡ *Harry Conquers His Addiction to Tobacco with Self-Hypnosis.* Harry consumed from two to three packages of cigarettes daily. He had learned about hypnosis being used to break habits, and he wanted to give up smoking altogether.

His father died at the age of 59 from lung cancer, and the family doctor had expressed the opinion that it may have been caused by excessive smoking. Harry had developed a chronic cough and was experiencing pains in the upper part of his chest. Although X-rays of his lungs were negative, he feared he, too, would someday develop lung cancer.

He wanted to learn about self-hypnosis. He was quite receptive and we taught Harry the 4-A's method of self-hypnosis described in Chapter 5. He suggested to himself that he would never smoke again or want to smoke again and that if he ever attempted to light a cigarette, he would break it in two.

Eighteen months have elapsed and Harry has not smoked since. He claims he has no desire to smoke and feels better physically and mentally knowing that he has been able to conquer a habit that has been worrying him for years.

⟼ *The Case of an Attorney Who Gave Up Chain Smoking Using Techniques of Hypnotic Self-Suggestion.* An attorney who had previously tried to stop smoking many times decided to put what he had just learned about self-hypnosis to the test. He describes his successful triumph over tobacco as follows:

> I first began to smoke when I was 17 years old. I have been smoking for the past 38 years. I started with 10 cigarettes a day and gradually increased to a point within the last two years of not being able to do anything without a cigarette or a cigar dangling from the corner of my mouth. I became a chain smoker. I smoked two to three packages of cigarettes a day, three or four cigars daily, and occasionally a pipe. I smoked before breakfast, during meals, between meals, and before going to sleep. It began to worry me. It got so bad that I was even talking to people with a cigarette in my mouth.
>
> It wasn't until I began to complain about a chronic cough, sore throat, and needlelike pains over my heart that I suspected these symptoms were caused by my excessive smoking. To confirm my suspicions, I consulted my doctor, who not only recommended that I stop smoking but warned me that my complaints would become worse and that I was risking the development of a serious heart dis-

order because of excessive nicotine in my system. I knew all the while that smoking wasn't good for me, yet it was difficult to stop. I know also that I would never be able to smoke in moderation. I had to make a decision. It was either quitting altogether or putting up with my symptoms and risking the consequences.

After many unsuccessful attempts to break the habit, I decided to try self-hypnosis. I had read several articles about how self-hypnosis had helped people to lose weight and had helped others who had a drinking problem and I decided that it could help me conquer my tobacco habit.

I subjected myself to being hypnotized, and in this way I learned to experience the feeling of relaxation. I concluded that I was using the pressures and problems at the office as excuses for my excessive smoking. I had developed the habit of chronic tension. I was unable to work in a relaxed way. There was no frustration at home in my relationship to my wife or my children, and the only thing that I could attribute my compulsion to smoke to excess was tension at work. I gave myself the posthypnotic suggestions that were recommended and learned to practice and apply the technique of self-hypnosis at home and at the office. I gave myself a session every morning before going to work for about three weeks and found that each day I was learning to enjoy working at the office without the old feeling of tension.

I had stopped smoking completely after my fourth session of self-hypnosis. In subsequent sessions I reinforced the suggestions I had given myself previously, and after three weeks I no longer needed to continue using self-hypnosis. My desire for any form of tobacco vanished. My symptoms also disappeared, and I have felt better than I have in a long time. I was worried that I would find a substitute outlet in excessive eating, but this has not been the case. In my autosuggestions I told myself that I would not resort to excessive eating to make up for not smoking.

Here are some of the self-suggestions I used to conquer my chain-smoking habit:

I have definitely made up my mind to stop smoking *completely*.
I am a nonsmoker.
I am proud to be a nonsmoker.

I am able to say "No thank you" whenever I am offered a cigarette or cigar.

I am going to enjoy better health as a result of being a nonsmoker.

I feel more confident knowing that I can do almost anything once I have made up my mind.

I no longer desire a cigarette or cigar because I am a nonsmoker.

I am convinced that becoming a nonsmoker will add years to my life.

My body feels better every day as a nonsmoker.

I am calm, relaxed, and breathing freely. I feel wonderful.

The Problem of Alcoholism and Other Addictions

When does a social drinker become an alcoholic? Drinking is a very complicated and individuated problem. One woman becomes violent after her first glass of wine. A young man goes on a systematic eight-day binge every 60 days. Another man drinks a pint of vodka every morning in his home. A 30-something woman starts drinking every Friday evening and continues drinking until Sunday morning, at which time she starts to "sleep it off" until Monday morning, when she goes back to her office job. Each of these people may be classified as alcoholics.

Not every drinker becomes an alcoholic. Some people can drink anytime they want to and stop when they please. Others lose control of their intake, and consequently they lose control of their lives.

Subconscious Causes of Excessive Drinking

There are several theories of why some people develop the compulsive urge to drink.

Most alcoholics are oversensitive and consequently are unable to withstand the frustrations of life. They are unable to discipline themselves sufficiently to give up drinking. Practically all suffer from an inferiority complex, which they try to drown out with alcohol.

Escapism is another theoretical explanation for excessive drinking. There are many normal people who dislike getting up in the morning and having to go to work. However, most of us realize that we can't escape our responsibilities.

Alcoholics seem to want to escape all of life's painful realities. They refuse to admit that through their own efforts and determination they can successfully overcome the normal problems of adult life, though all about them they may see other people doing so. They see themselves as "different."

There are various methods of escaping reality. Some gamble, while others become philanderers. Some use drugs, and still others prefer alcohol. The underlying motive, however, is the same, to anesthetize or assuage the mental pain caused by personal misfortunes.

Unpaid debts, an unhappy marriage, failure in business, and physical illness all constitute surface alibis for excessive drinking. The real truth is that the victims of alcoholism have a difficult time enduring the common adversities of life.

Yet another theory is that alcoholism represents a vicarious or *disguised form of self-destruction.*

Many psychiatrists are of the opinion that alcoholics are people who commit what might be termed "psychological suicide." They die a slow death, only because they are unable to recognize the true motive that unconsciously inspires their sense of defeat—their hopelessness.

Alcohol addiction becomes the compromise between the wish to live and a wish to die. It is a partial suicide—a "poisoning" of the body and mind but usually not enough to cause death. The alcoholic lives and dies at will, too scared to die and too afraid to live. *He or she lives in a third world.*

Still another explanation why some people drink to excess is for the *release of inhibitions.*

We all have primitive emotions for which we secretly crave an outlet. But we cannot give way to them because our sober conscious mind will not permit.

A man may be too inhibited to show his affection for his girl-friend. From his outward behavior you would assume that he is a "perfect gentleman." But deep inside he wishes he had the courage to put his arm around his girl and profess his love for her. Liquid stimulants loosen his tongue. Alcohol makes him the "Casanova" he wishes to be in real life. He becomes expansive and witty as well as romantic only because he now has an excuse for his bold behavior. If he is rebuffed he can always blame it on that "one cocktail too many."

As Dr. Walter Miles stated: "Alcohol unburdens the individual of his cares and fears, relieves him of his feelings of inferiority and weakness. The inhibitions and self-criticism which ordinarily cramp his feelings tend, after alcohol, to be put aside."

The Treatment of Alcoholism

Many forms of treatment for the alcoholic exist. Alcoholics Anonymous uses self-examination and honesty. It has by far the most impressive rate of success of any other form of treatment. Transactional Analysis isolates the "crazy child" and alters his or her behavior. Psychotherapy searches for roots in dependency and the symbolic meaning of the bottle. Allopathic medicine often prescribes drugs that cause vomiting to occur when alcohol is ingested. The nausea causes an aversion reaction that, in turn, modifies the behavior. All of these systems work for some, and none of them work for all.

Self-Hypnosis Can Help

Self-hypnosis is a tool that can be effective in overcoming alcoholism, especially if it is used in conjunction with participation in an AA program and/or professional counseling. You can use the auto-analysis part of your self-hypnosis session to understand the psychological factors responsible for your addiction to alcohol. As we have said before, knowledge is power.

During this time of probing for answers, trace your habit back to its root cause in light of what you have just learned about why some people drink to excess. Ask yourself a lot of questions. Study your answers when you think you have discovered the subconscious reasons for your drinking and then provide the self-suggestions you need.

The following can serve as a sample of what you might tell yourself. You can also make up your own, more personalized suggestions. Repeat them out loud or silently during as many sessions as you may require:

1. I can survive life's frustrations without alcohol.

2. I choose to abstain from drinking.

3. By giving up alcohol, I am rewarded by feeling better physically and mentally.

4. I am self-sufficient. I abstain because I *want* to.

5. Each day that I abstain is a day closer to successful permanent abstinence.

6. I remind myself of the things I have learned and now understand through autoanalysis (the subconscious reasons for my excessive drinking).

7. I find healthier outlets for personal frustrations that arise from day to day.

8. I practice self-hypnosis so that I can relax myself without external aids.

9. I am a nondrinker.

10. I shall repeat this over and over again during sessions of self-hypnosis.

11. I will avail myself of help from Alcoholics Anonymous if need be.

➥ *Case of Compulsive Drinking That Responded Successfully to Self-Hypnosis.*   George was a bachelor architect who worked long hours. He would end his day's work by retreating to his apartment and drinking a pint of whiskey every evening. Gradually, this was increased to one or two fifths over the weekends, and he soon found that he was unable to work during the day unless he had a "few drinks." He felt compelled to drink—a beginning symptom of dipsomania (craving for alcohol).

His practice began to deteriorate. He disappointed his clients and developed an indifference toward everything. Nothing seemed to interest him. He withdrew more and more into himself.

Finally, he decided he was going to try self-hypnosis. Much to his own amazement, after his third session he stopped drinking. He informs us that now he is able to work without tension and is able to lose himself in his recreational hobby on weekends.

Drug Addiction

Unfortunately, insidious habits can take many faces. In addition to the millions of people plagued by excessive smoking and drinking, millions more are ensnared by the addiction to drugs. According to the World Health Organization, "Drug addiction is a state of periodic and chronic intoxication detrimental to the individual and to society, produced by the repeated consumption of a natural or synthetic drug. Characteristics of addiction include: (1) An overpowering desire to continue use; (2) An emotional drive to obtain it by any means; (3) A tendency to increase the dose as the drug lessens its powers; (4) A psychological and sometimes physical dependence."

This definition includes over-the-counter drugs, prescription drugs, and illegal street drugs.

Addictions and Addictive Thinking

Addicts of all kinds seem to share similar beliefs whether the addiction is to alcohol or to drugs. Some of the common beliefs of addicts are:

I am separate from everybody else.

I am different.

My situation is different.

In order for me to feel safe, I must judge others.

For me to feel good, I have to be right.

For me to feel good, I have to be perfect

Guilt is a part of life.

I am a victim of circumstance.

Mistakes must be punished.

Unless you like me, I have no self-worth.

I can control another person's behavior.

I am in a cruel world, and I am alone.

Other people's actions are responsible for my feelings.

Do you recognize any of these feelings as your own? Are there others you can think of that are in the same general category?

Self-Hypnosis and Drugs

Drug addiction may be effectively treated with self-hypnosis as long as your motivation is real and you are diligent with your practice sessions. We strongly recommend that you also participate in a 12-step program (such as AA or NA) to reinforce the benefits of self-hypnosis. Drug addiction is a difficult problem to overcome. People who deny that are fooling themselves. However, research has shown that the presence of certain factors in your life greatly increases your probability of success. You can begin your personal self-hypnosis program by creating the presence of these elements in your own life.

What Does It Take to Quit?

- *You must believe you can do it.* As soon as you have the absolute belief that you can quit your addiction, you are on the road to success. Believing that you can quit on your own is one of the most important factors in your overall success. You must recognize that the ultimate responsibility is yours, and no one outside yourself can do this for you.

- *Design your own personalized program.* When you take responsibility for the structure of your own program, your sense of self-sufficiency increases. With every small success, it increases even more. This increases your belief and reinforces the first point.

- *Learn how to interpret failure.* Remember that you did not become an addict overnight; be patient with yourself. If the program you design does not work the first time, "fine-tune" it and try again. People who succeed recognize that the flaw is in the program, not in themselves.

- *Value health.* When you value being healthy, you are less inclined to let drugs or alcohol control your life.

- *Develop interests in new activities.* When you value your family, your work, or any other activity you do, you will refrain from abusing your body with drugs. When you fill your life with activities you cherish, you will have no interest in altering your consciousness with abusive substances.

Through the 4-A's method of self-hypnosis, you can become more optimistic. You will discover within yourself the ability to make your life better. The great treasure of inner peace and tranquility that comes from knowing that you are a healthy, balanced person who makes a positive contribution to life is within the reach of your own mind.

Suggestions That Will Assist You in Designing Your Personalized Program

Start by reviewing the suggestions we gave you in the previous section on alcoholism. Since the addictions to alcohol and drugs are so psychologically similar, you can easily adapt most of those suggestions to apply to quitting drugs. Then look over the following list and choose the ones that are most meaningful for you personally.

This is the most important thing I can do for my life and my health.

I see my body as healthy and whole.

I look for the best in everyone.

Nothing is more important than my health.

I lovingly accept myself.

I am interested in others.

I enjoy my new energy and vitality.

I am an honest person.

As my body detoxifies, I feel better and better.

I am so proud of myself for my accomplishments.

I control what goes into my body.

I consume healthful, nutritious food.

I value my body.

Because I depend on my body for my existence, I treat it with loving care.

I see the truth.

I speak the truth.

I choose health and wholeness.

Chapter 9

The Hypnotic Road to Restful Sleep

If you are like most other people, you have experienced nights when you tossed and turned, finally falling asleep just moments before you have to get up. It seemed that the harder you tried to fall asleep, the wider awake you became. Nearly everyone has had such a problem at one time or another. According to data from the American Sleep Disorders Association, nearly 30 million Americans suffer from insomnia at some time in their lives.

How Much Sleep Is Enough?

We all must have regular sleep, but all of us have different sleep requirements. What may be considered a good night's sleep for one person may be entirely inadequate for another. Some are fine with four or five hours of sleep; others require eight or ten. Your body will determine what is right for you. It seems that as we grow older, we require less sleep. A baby sleeps off and on night and day, and adults average between six and eight hours. You should get enough sleep to feel refreshed and vigorous throughout the next day.

121

Many Factors Cause Sleeplessness

Here are just a few of them:

- *Taking worrisome troubles to bed with you.* You cannot expect to get a good night's sleep if you lie awake worrying about your work or some problem in your life. Many people have the tendency to try to solve their dilemma by thinking about them. Such challenges do require thinking in order to be solved, but it is unlikely that the solving will occur during an anxious, restless night. Self-hypnosis can help you break the habit of thinking too much at bedtime.

- *Being obsessed with the false idea that you just can't sleep.* Labeling yourself as an "insomniac" is just giving yourself a negative suggestion. You begin to believe it, and it becomes true. Self-hypnosis can help you reverse your thinking on this.

- *Tension and/or fatigue.* Going to bed feeling overfatigued may cause you to have a sleepless night. Often when you are overtired, your body is very tense. When you go to bed, even though you feel exhausted, your body tenses up, and you can't fall asleep. Self-hypnosis will provide you with the means to relax completely every time you go to bed.

- *Pain and discomfort from an illness.* If your mind is focused on the object of your pain or discomfort, it is not going to be willing to shut itself down for rest. Whether your discomfort is a temporary one such as a sprained wrist or a chronic one such as arthritis, you can still rely on your new skills to come to your assistance. Self-hypnosis will help you to alleviate your discomfort.

- *Bad sleeping conditions.* Maybe your mattress is too hard. Perhaps a crying infant awakens you. Or a telephone call might disturb your sleep. Others find it impossible to sleep away from home. Poor ventilation, hot weather, cold weather, snoring partners, and many other things can disturb a night's sleep. Self-hypnosis will enable you to get your rest in spite of it all.

- *Guilt feelings.* If you go to bed with a "bad conscience," you may find it difficult to fall asleep. You worry about whatever it was that caused the bad feelings. Guilt causes fear, which brings on anxiety and insomnia. You can use self-hypnosis to help put your mind at ease.

- *Bad habits.* Eating or drinking too much right before bed will almost assure anyone of a restless night. The relaxation techniques of self-hypnosis are conducive to sleep.

➡ **When Charlotte Learned the Techniques of Self-Hypnosis, She No Longer Needed Sleeping Pills.** Charlotte's insomnia started just after the death of her widowed mother. Her mother died of cancer at the age of 56. Charlotte found herself thinking about her mother every night. She would often cry in her sleep. She became depressed, lost weight, and became obsessed with the fear that she would never be able to adjust to her grief. She was tense and nervous at work and unable to get herself interested in anything recreational.

Charlotte was assured that she could learn how to attain the hypnotic state and relax, that if she once developed the ability to relax her body and her mind every night she would eventually be able to sleep well and would no longer have to take sleeping pills.

Many patients suffering from a distressing health symptom will do anything for relief. Charlotte was amenable to the idea of being hypnotized and became a good hypnotic subject. She went into a state of relaxation quickly and responded favorably to suggestive therapy. Our next task was to teach her the technique of self-hypnosis so that she could relax at home and in bed and sleep soundly through the night. We gave her the same instructions as described under the technique of self-relaxation in Chapter 5. She would repeat such phrases as

My eyes are getting very tired—very tired. Soon I will close my eyes and sleep will come.

My body is becoming more and more relaxed.

I feel all my muscles relaxing.

I am getting sleepier and sleepier and sleepier.

As I count backwards very slowly and silently starting with 100–99–98, etc., I will go into a deeper and deeper and deeper state of relaxation.

Soon the numbers will disappear, and I will fall fast asleep.

When I awaken in the morning, I will feel refreshed and will have had a wonderful night's sleep.

She practiced these self-suggestions and discovered that after a week's time she was able to fall asleep without having to count.

➠ *A Case of Insomnia Caused by Feelings of Guilt.* Laura, the mother of three children, consulted her doctor because of her recent inability to sleep. As a consequence of many nights of sleeplessness she lost weight, developed a tremor of her hands, and was unable to work because of fatigue and general lassitude. Her doctor began to suspect her problem of insomnia was caused by emotional conflicts and recommended a psychiatric evaluation of her case.

Laura began using techniques of self-hypnosis, and during one of her self-analytic sessions she became aware that she had been indulging in fantasies that produced feelings of guilt, which accounted for her insomnia.

"I shouldn't be thinking of such things," she said. "I feel I'm being unfaithful to my husband. I can't seem to get this certain man out of my mind. It keeps me awake."

She was greatly relieved when told that she need not feel too responsible or guilty and that the less she worried, the sooner she would be able to sleep. She gave herself the following post-hypnotic suggestion.

"I can and will fall asleep. I am using self-hypnosis to relax my body and my mind. My thoughts are my own and harmful to no one. I am comfortable with my thoughts. I fall asleep without difficulty."

How to Induce Restful Sleep

1. Get into the habit of going to bed at approximately the same hour each night.

2. Make sure conditions are conducive to good sleeping.

3. Practice the technique of autorelaxation 15 minutes each night.

4. Remind yourself that tension causes insomnia and now that you are relaxing your whole body and your mind, tension will quickly disappear as you master the art of relaxation.

5. Tell yourself that you can sleep—that you will soon fall asleep—that you are feeling sleepier and sleepier.

6. Lie still in bed and avoid as much as possible unnecessary tossing and changing of position.

7. Keep your eyes closed and repeat to yourself that you are becoming more and more relaxed, that sleep will soon come.

8. Look forward to going to bed. Don't worry about not being able to sleep

9. Use soft music if you find it helps to relax you.

10. Think pleasant thoughts, thoughts that are conducive to sleeping well. Relive in your sleep experiences that you enjoyed. Keep your thoughts positive.

Some Self-Hypnotic Exercises for Restful Sleep

Notice the way your body feels in your bed. Become aware of the weight of your body on the mattress as you tense and relax your muscles from head to toe. Feel the tension in your body melting away, leaving you relaxed and comfortable. Breathe deeply, telling yourself that each breath is making you drowsier and drowsier.

Visualize yourself in a hammock, swinging back and forth, side to side, getting sleepier and sleepier.

Picture yourself in a little boat, floating on a calm lake.

See yourself reclining in a comfortable recliner, looking out a picture window at a peaceful pastoral scene. Watch the clouds as they drift slowly by and notice the patterns they form.

Count backwards slowly from one hundred to zero.

Self-Hypnosis Leads You to Sleep Naturally

The fact that self-hypnosis causes you to relax on the brink of sleep makes it a very reliable tool to use for insomnia. It is a safe, natural way to find a long-term solution for your sleepless nights. You deserve to enjoy the benefits of a restful sleep every night. The adequate sleep essential to good health can be yours with self-hypnosis.

C h a p t e r
10

What Self-Hypnosis Can Do to Make Your Sex Life More Exciting

Sexual fulfillment is a complex phenomenon, an intricately woven human event that is comprised of emotional, mental, and physical responses. It is important to realize that both men and women have sexual-functioning problems at times. In either gender, a problem usually occurs when there is *mental* interference—and that leads to emotional insecurity. It is therefore sensible to assume that hypnosis can play an important role in the alleviation or correction of sexual dysfunction or dissatisfaction since sexual problems are most likely to be rooted in emotional or mental issues. In order for you to use self-hypnosis for assistance in solving your sexual problem, you must approach it in exactly the same way you approach any other issue.

Sexual deprivation and dysfunction are habits that are learned behavior. They can be unlearned, replaced with self-fulfilling habits. Some people go though life sexually unfulfilled with relationships rife with tension and low expectations. Don't let this dismal portrayal be you. The requirement of self-actualization is a basic human need, and an emotionally and physically satisfying sex life is part of that requirement.

Self-Love: The Most Important Element

You are undoubtedly a better lover than you think you are. The first recipient of this love must be yourself. Allow yourself to experience an abundance of self-appreciation by using your self-hypnosis skills. This self-love is absolutely necessary if you want to have a truly satisfying sex life with someone else.

Avoidance of Sex

One of the most common problems at the root of sexual inadequacy in both males and females is fatigue. Sometimes it's real; other times it's imagined. Believe it or not, contrary to the popular jokes about women and their headaches, the excuse is as common among men as women. Some become mentally exhausted when they think about sex, which may be a result of a fear of failure of some kind. Others, because of whatever is their emotional problem with sex, come to consider having sex to be a burden of obligation instead of a source of pleasure.

For women, lack of sexual response may be a complicated issue. It may be rooted in fear: fear of pain, fear of rejection, fear of pregnancy, and/or fear of sexually transmitted disease. Many women are so uncomfortable with their sexual selves that they suppress their natural sexual desires and build up tremendous amounts of tension. This tension ultimately manifests itself in some physical ailment.

➦ *Mary's Problem of Frigidity.*   Mary claimed she was in love with her husband, but despite how much she loved him she was unable to achieve an orgasm. She consulted two gynecologists who assured her there was no physical condition to account for her problem. She thought at first that it was congenital, that perhaps some women just didn't have any feeling or sensation in the vagina and that it was best to try to become reconciled to this fact and not worry about it. This is what she had been told by some of her friends who confessed to her that they had the same problem.

Consequently, the first thing that had to be done was to make her realize that she had been *misinformed*, that frigidity is not congenital. We told her also that frigidity is subconscious and that it can be helped with self-hypnosis. She was excited. We informed her that frigidity is a complex symptom, the result of some one or more factors in the past and that these contributing influences could be recalled with hypnosis. We assured her that once she began to understand why and how her frigidity developed, she would be able to adopt a new attitude toward sex and be able to relax and achieve sexual satisfaction. Incidentally, this latter information was given to her while she was in a state of hypnotic relaxation.

After one or two preliminary sessions of hypnosis, at a given word signal she was able to induce her own hypnotic state of relaxation. She had practiced at home the various suggestibility tests mentioned in this book and was anxious to begin her session of autoanalysis.

EXPERIENCES FROM HER PAST. Mary recalled an experience that occurred when she was ten years old. She was on her way home from school when she saw a man open his trousers behind a tree and call to her. She became frightened and ran home to tell her mother. She remembers her mother reporting the incident to the police over the telephone. Afterward, her mother told her that men did bad and ugly things. During her high-school years a girl once kissed her on the lips. Nothing else happened, but she remembered feeling kind of "funny" about it. When she learned about homosexuality in later years, she worried, thinking she had homosexual tendencies. She has had occasional dreams of a homosexual nature. At the age of 19, she was raped by a cousin. She told her mother about it. Her mother had her examined by a physician and was relieved when she was told she was not pregnant.

At her home, during subsequent sessions of self-analysis in a hypnotic state, she remembered that whenever she had relations with her husband she was unable to relax. She felt "unclean." She associated sex with something she had to endure rather than enjoy. She felt "held back." She loved her husband, enjoyed being kissed by him, but when he began the sex act, something happened to her. She couldn't bring herself around to participating in the love play—"I turned to stone. I felt nothing. I would tell my husband not to wait for me."

HOW SELF-HYPNOSIS SOLVED MARY'S PROBLEMS.   We put into writing
for her a few suggestions she could repeat to herself during autohypnosis sessions at home, suggestions such as:

> I have gained a better understanding of my problem. I am a
> warm person, and sex is an expression of love.
>
> I am more enthusiastic and active during lovemaking with my
> husband.
>
> I close my eyes and concentrate on the pleasurable sensations
> I am experiencing during sex.
>
> I am sexually healthy and normal.
>
> I relax and allow the orgasm to occur.
>
> I abandon myself during the sex act and experience a feeling
> of "total sexual surrender." Whatever a husband and wife do to
> express their love for each other is normal and good.
>
> I achieve an orgasm whenever I want.

Mary has succeeded in getting sexual satisfaction. She attributes her success to her complete change of attitude about sex, to the
fact that she developed confidence in herself through self-hypnosis,
believing that she would reach a climax. She says that the insight
into the cause of her frigidity helped immensely and that the self-
given suggestions—that sex was something to be enjoyed, that it is
an expression of love—enabled her to relax and achieve orgasms.

We hope that the many thousands of other women who are disturbed and frustrated because of this same problem will be encouraged to put self-hypnosis to the test. One thing we know—it cannot
do harm. It can only do good. Self-hypnosis is bound to *improve*
your sex life. If you doubt this, try it.

➠ *Another Case Illustration of a Sexual-Frustration Problem
Solved with Self-Hypnosis.*   Here is Maureen's description in her
own words of how she applied self-hypnosis to improve her sex life
and achieve sexual satisfaction.

> For me, the most difficult part of achieving an orgasm was convinc-
> ing myself that it was a possibility. I could not do this, and it was not

for want of desire or for effort spent. If a woman has spent five years having sex, experiencing various positions and moods, reading between 15 and 20 sex manuals, and still has had no results, she obviously must seek help elsewhere. I was such a woman.

My biggest mistake was waiting until I was so buried in failure and frustration that I was positive that even if there was hope for every other frigid woman in the whole world, there was none for me. It was in this frame of mind that I went to see Dr. Caprio.

He taught me to relax and to have faith and confidence in myself. He taught me that I was not different, that I was as capable of enjoying sex as any other woman. He taught me to suggest these things to myself at home.

Gradually, the ideas began to penetrate, and I began to have a more positive outlook not just on sex, but on life itself. I went to a gynecologist to be sure I was getting any necessary medical help. Gradually, I became a better sex partner, and I began getting results.

For me, it was a matter of saying over and over, "Yes, I can. I know I can." This is how self-hypnosis worked for me. If you tell yourself enough times, you will believe it, and if you believe it, it will happen. And if it happened for me, it can happen for anyone.

The Use of Self-Hypnosis for the Problem of Impotence

Fears are not the exclusive purview of women, mind you. Behind a man's complaint of being exhausted may also lie repressed fears. Men's greatest sexual fear—by far—is the fear of failure to perform, the fear of impotence. This means the inability to get and sustain an erection long enough to satisfy his partner. It is a widely held belief among the experts in human sexuality that in the vast majority of cases, a man's impotency is psychological rather than physical.

Impotence is an all encompassing term for sexual inadequacy in the male. Like frigidity in women, there are various types of impotence in men. Inability to become sexually aroused, failure to carry out the sex act, lack of sexual desire, and premature ejaculation are only a few of the many kinds of impotence reactions.

Autoanalysis will often reveal the causative emotional factors responsible for the development of this sexual disorder. In questioning yourself during a session of self-analysis, keep in mind the following factors that can cause you to experience difficulty in achieving sexual fulfillment: sexual ignorance, inhibitory influences, sexual bashfulness, fear, guilt feelings, insecurity, fear of sexually transmitted disease, faulty attitudes toward sex, homosexual conflicts, fear of making a woman pregnant, fear of causing a woman pain, dislike of contraceptives, fear of being seen or interrupted during the sex act, and numerous other causes.

Ask yourself if your impotence is caused by some specific frustration involving your partner. If it is, discuss the matter with her and enlist her cooperation. Use auto-reconditioning to make yourself less sensitive. Letting little things bother you can diminish your sexual potency.

Understanding the specific cause of impotence makes it easier to respond successfully to self-hypnosis.

First, you must rule out *physical* causes. Your doctor is the best qualified person to tell you if your impotence is caused by a condition that requires medical treatment. As was mentioned earlier, in the majority of cases, impotence is due to *psychological* causes.

Self-hypnosis can prove very effective in removing mental blocks responsible for sexual inadequacy. It can restore your confidence in your ability to perform. Your posthypnotic suggestions must be along the lines of removing fears, having confidence in your technique of lovemaking, knowing that you are going to enjoy the sex act, and that you are in command of your own feelings and attitudes. The repetition of these thoughts under a self-induced hypnotic state paves the way toward restoring your potency.

⟶ *Harold Finally Solved His Sexual Problem with Self-Hypnosis.* Some husbands use the male menopause as an excuse for their loss of interest in sexual relations. Our patient Harold developed neurotic health ailments that he used as an alibi for his sexual apathy or indifference. When the health symptoms are subjective in origin and have no organic basis, the condition is psychosomatic.

Harold began calling his doctor, telling him that he suffered from indigestion, irritability, and general nervousness. His doctor found nothing wrong with him physically. Harold continued to complain of tension and thought that he was about to suffer a nervous breakdown, attributing it to overwork. Actually, he had little responsibility at work and plenty of time for relaxation in the evenings. Inquiring into his sex life, we learned that Harold had a tendency to deny any connection between his sex life and the way he felt physically. He stated: "My sex life is all right. Of course, I don't have sexual relations with my wife as frequently as I did, but I have no conflicts about my diminished virility."

As soon as Harold learned techniques of self-hypnosis, which he began to put into practice, he learned that he was not really suffering from the fear of a nervous breakdown, but from the fear of impotence, and that his health complaints were but a manifestation of his anxiety concerning his potency. Realizing this, he began to change for the better. He assured himself during self-hypnosis that potency is a matter of mental attitude. He resumed regular sexual relations, and his symptoms began to disappear.

Start with an Inventory of Your Sex Life

After you have induced a state of hypnotic self-relaxation, concentrate on your specific sexual problem, assuming you have one. Ask yourself a series of questions. In answering them during your self-analysis stage of autohypnosis, try to develop some understanding of your particular sexual issue. You will surprise yourself as to how much self insight you will gain this way, insight that will enable you to find the solution to your problem.

When you've recognized and defined your problem, you're well on your way to solving it. For example, if you are aware of having a faulty attitude about sex because of some neurotic parental influence, tell yourself that you can and will develop a healthier, more positive attitude. If you are living in the past, tormenting yourself with guilt feelings because of some past sexual transgression, accept the self-hypnosis suggestion that you are going to close the door to the past, forgive yourself, and live in the present.

Questions to Ask Yourself

1. Do I harbor guilt feelings about some past sexual experience that is interfering with my sex life now?
2. Am I handicapped by my lack of knowledge about sex?
3. Is sexual incompatibility the basic cause of my relationship problems?
4. Am I sexually immature?
5. Do I really enjoy the sex act and achieve sexual satisfaction?
6. Do I have a puritanical attitude toward sex?
7. Is my lack of sexual satisfaction due to conventional shame and crippling inhibitions?
8. Do I have a specific sexual difficulty that needs to be addressed?
9. Is my attitude toward sex being appropriately conveyed to my partner?
10. Am I a responsive lover?

You may think of many more questions of your own that are more appropriate to your personal situation.

Twenty-one Suggestions to Give Yourself in Autotherapy

1. I enjoy lovemaking.
2. I have fulfillment each time I participate in lovemaking.
3. Sex is healthy and proper.
4. I am guilt-free.
5. I openly discuss sexual matters with my partner.
6. I am comfortable with my body.
7. I enjoy learning about sex.

8. My relationship with my partner is strengthened by our sexual intimacy.

9. My love relationship is a reciprocal one.

10. I enjoy a healthy sexual relationship.

11. I am unencumbered by anything that keeps me from achieving orgasm.

12. I am an adult with adult reasoning.

13. Sex is a relaxed, natural process.

14. I am responsible for my feelings.

15. I enjoy a new patience with myself and with my partner.

16. My body responds easily and naturally.

17. I am enjoying my new attitude of sexual freedom and responsibility.

18. I am thinking more clearly about life and love.

19. As my partner touches me, I become relaxed and responsive.

20. The desire for sex is a natural human response.

21. I am pleased with my sexuality.

Confronting and correcting sexual problems is of prime importance in any relationship. If these problems are left to grow, hostilities develop that can destroy a relationship. Problems in the bedroom have an insidious way of spreading out to involve and disrupt the other areas of your life.

Self-hypnosis is a powerful tool for helping you with your sex life. In the autoanalysis phase of your session, you can recall the past conditioning that has led to your current sexual problems. When you have that understanding, it becomes a relatively simple matter for you to reprogram your subconscious mind so that you can truly enjoy sex.

Chapter 11

Overcome Tension, Chronic Tiredness, and Pain with Self-Hypnosis

Every thought and every experience you have contains a feeling. It is impossible for you to think about or to do anything without a feeling of some kind.

⇒ *A Case Study of Tension Reactions.* About a year ago we encountered a most unusual experience that entailed both hypnosis and autohypnosis. A young man who had been referred to us by someone we had helped called long distance and asked if we could give him a session of hypnosis over the telephone. He explained that he was on his way to a university to report for an oral examination, one of the requirements he had to meet before he could receive his master's degree. He had completed his thesis, and it had been approved and accepted. He had fulfilled all his other requirements. However, he kept postponing the date for his oral examination, in which he would have to "defend" his thesis by answering whatever questions were put to him by a group of faculty members.

He panicked at the thought of having to face those examiners. "What if I make a bad showing?" "What if my mind goes blank?" "What if I get nervous and am unable to give them the kind of an answer they want?" These and many other thoughts plagued him. He realized he couldn't go on putting off what he had to face someday if he wanted his M.A. degree, something he had worked very hard for.

Prior to calling us, he committed himself to a definite date and so informed the faculty. As the time for his departure approached, he became more and more tense and apprehensive. For several nights he had tossed in bed wondering what they were going to ask him. He began to have doubts as to whether he was adequately prepared for the ordeal. Nevertheless, he was determined to go through with it this time. He had read about hypnosis and was eager to be helped. It was impossible, so he claimed, to come to Washington for his session. Not having any alternative, we agreed to try it by phone.

We began by explaining that all hypnosis is really self-hypnosis, that he had to teach himself to eliminate tension and conquer what he termed "anticipatory anxiety" (the fear that not all may go well—a fear of the worst happening). We consoled him by informing him he was not alone with his problem, that many individuals go through this panic-like state just before making a speech or taking an examination or doing anything that is tension producing. We further consoled him by stating that this panic or anxiety state before an examination could definitely be conquered by the individual himself, that he had it in his powers to reduce tension to its minimum, which would enable him to do relaxed and clear thinking.

We then proceeded to explain over the phone in a separate session the technique of self-relaxation, how to practice increasing his receptivity to suggestion so that he would accept his own positive thoughts. We suggested that in his self-analysis sessions he try to analyze why he feared taking his orals and why he thought he would fail them. Was he fully prepared? Had he studied enough? Did he think the professors wanted to flunk him deliberately? Was he afraid of one particular examiner? In other words, we suggested that he try to ferret out the root cause of his anxiety. Our last instruction was to have him write down a list of positive suggestions he was going to give himself and to repeat them en route to the university until he believed everything he needed to believe.

Upon his return, he told us it wasn't half as bad as he had anticipated. He admitted beforehand to his examiners that he was a bit nervous, but that he had studied hard and hoped that he would pass. They treated him with all the sympathy and consideration they could give him. He was later notified that he had passed. His experience with autohypnosis has inspired him to apply the technique he learned to his daily life, particularly when he is confronted with any kind of fear-producing situation.

Attitudes Are Habitual

This may sound a bit far-fetched at first, but since we know that the same kind of feeling can appear with very different experiences, we begin to understand how attitudes and moods are formed. Consider this hypothetical example:

Suppose you are a person who enjoys eating good food at nice restaurants. You read in your local paper that a fine restaurant chain is planning to open one in your town. *You feel happy*. Later, you find out that the location of the new restaurant is to be very convenient to your home. *You feel happy*. As the building progresses, you can see that the restaurant is going to be a beautiful place, a credit to the community. *You feel happy*. The landscaping is lovely, colorful, and a pleasure to view. *You feel happy*. You are among the first to try the restaurant on opening night, and the ambiance delights you. The lighting and music are perfect. *You feel happy*. When the menu arrives and you observe the interesting, delectable dishes, you are thrilled, and *you feel happy*. By this time, you have had many instances of feeling "happy" regarding this restaurant. The result is that you have a happy attitude about it because that feeling has been repeated often enough to have become a habit without your even realizing it. Attitudes are feelings that have become habits. Unfortunately, this is true of unpleasant feelings as well as pleasant ones.

Tension Becomes a Habit

Yes, it's true. Tension often does become a habit and results in self-limiting and self-defeating behavior. We live active, demanding lives. Often we encounter events that we perceive as threats or dangers. Sometimes our expectations aren't met, and we are left dissatisfied. We frequently overextend ourselves with multiple commitments and tasks, creating a day-to-day life that is little more than a perpetual cycle of tension and fatigue.

Whatever the origin, tension becomes a habit. If a variety of situations makes you tense, and the tension is repeated in each situation, you will invariably incorporate tension as an integral part of your overall demeanor. You may even consider tension as a natural state for yourself. Your family and friends may describe you as "high-strung." You may be completely unaware what it is like to relax and enjoy yourself.

Tension Breeds Psychosomatic Difficulties

Some of the many physical complaints that can have psychosomatic origins include ulcers, gastric dysfunction, skin disorders, allergies, asthma, and headaches, just to name a few.

It has been known for centuries that there is an important relationship between the mind and the body. In recent years, this important, intimate connection is being recognized by established medicine and psychology. One of the pioneers of this movement is Dr. Carl Simonton of California whose groundbreaking work, *Getting Well Again*, describes how he taught his cancer patients to use visualization to ease the discomfort of chemotherapy and to actually combat their disease. Other notable physicians who have joined in the mind/body movement are Bernie Siegel, M.D., Deepak Chopra, M.D, and Joan Borysenko, M.D. A partial listing of their books is in the references section. We strongly recommend any and all of them.

Tension Breeds Fatigue

Some fatigue is normal. Every human being becomes tired. Normal fatigue is a protective device, forcing us to rest. Nature takes care of this normal tiredness through the revitalizing mechanism of sleep. During sleep, our bodies rest and become refreshed. Fatigue disappears.

There is, however, another type of tiredness that is chronic and exaggerated. It exhibits itself in the feeling of being "born tired." It is the result of a mind/body reaction or state caused by constant tension, negative thinking, and anger. People who are angry or disappointed often go through the entire day with clenched jaws and tensed muscles, particularly their shoulders and neck. It's no wonder they feel tired.

It's not the amount of work you do, but the manner in which you do that work that's tiring. Don't try to crowd into a single day more tasks than you can reasonably accomplish well. Budget your energy. Don't work an excess number of hours.

Is Your Work "Working" for You?

Working at a job you dislike or for which you are not suited also makes you tired. If you must continue at this work because of its financial compensation or because no other job is available, then you must develop some interest outside work that you thoroughly enjoy. If you have a sedentary job, plan an "active" activity. If you must be in motion all day at your job, enjoy your leisure hours by listening to a concert, reading a book, or some other restful, rewarding activity.

We have had patients who claim they would actually gag and become nauseated every morning just thinking about having to go to work. Their attitude was a totally negative one. They disliked their jobs, complained about their aches and pains, and experienced boredom because of the monotony of day-to-day living. Every day was viewed as a battle to be won. This kind of struggle was sure to bring on exaggerated tiredness. In truth, they were simply victims of emotionally induced fatigue. They were basically unhappy, just tired of life. In each case, we taught these people the 4-A's principles of self-hypnosis, and they all experienced positive changes in their lives. We know you can, too.

Own Your Attitudes and Habits

There is no question that we were taught or programmed to feel about certain things in certain ways by other people in our lives. It may have been in the form of deliberate direction from our parents or teachers. It may have occurred quite indirectly from our own experience in thousands of other, more subtle ways. Even a causal remark or a recurring thought may have resulted in the establishment of attitudes and feelings we have now.

Regardless of how you came to have your moods or attitudes, they are now yours; they belong to you. You own them. If, when you examine them you find them self-limiting and inappropriate, you can use your self-hypnosis skills to transform them to feelings that will bring you satisfaction and self-fulfillment.

A Feeling Analyzed Is a Feeling Owned

We've already explained that a feeling accompanies your every thought and every act. And now for an amazing fact. We also know that once feelings are noticed and analyzed, they tend to diminish in intensity . . . and as the feeling you are noticing begins to diminish in intensity, you will discover that the opposite feeling comes in to take its place.

If you want to see a demonstration of this fascinating phenomenon, you can do an experiment. The next time you have a group of friends at your house having a good time, pass out paper and pencils to them and ask them to write down the reasons they are enjoying themselves. They will inevitably groan and complain that you are spoiling the party. The very thought of analyzing their good feelings will result in the opposite feelings taking over.

Self-Hypnosis: Your Built-in Tranquilizer

With your self-hypnosis skills, you can relieve your tension and reprogram your attitudes. On the morning when you get up and feel unhappy at the prospect of facing the day, stop and take the time to do a self-hypnosis practice session. Don't start the day with trepidation. It is far better to get started a little late with a good attitude than to go off on time with an already-ruined day.

The Worry Habit: What Can You Do?

There are many aspects of worry that we have catalogued in our many years of practice. Here are a few of the things we have come to believe are generally true about worry.

1. Excessive worrying about anything is an acquired habit. Worry is not an inherited trait. If you are around worriers, you are inclined to develop the same habit. Parents who are fearful generally project their anxiety and fears onto their children. When the children grow up, they usually find themselves imitating their parents. Worry and negativity are contagious conditions. Don't get caught up in the imitation of someone else's neuroses.

2. Excessive worry solves nothing. Making yourself sick with worry only adds to your misery.

3. Chronic worrying is a symptom of insecurity—evidence of a lack of self-confidence.

4. The habit of worrying is just like any other habit. It can be conquered once you make the decision to change it.

5. Worry is fatigue producing and health destroying.

6. Use autoanalysis to understand the problem you are worried about.

7. Convert the energy you used for worrying into solving the problem. Doing something about it makes much more sense than worrying.

8. If you are worrying about something about which you have no control, you must let it go. *Let it go!*

9. Practice observing your thoughts. When you catch yourself worrying, mentally picture a STOP sign. Immediately begin thinking of something else. You *can* choose your thoughts.

10. As we've pointed out before, recognition of your problem is half the battle. When you know what you are fighting, the battle's almost won.

Twenty-five Examples of Self-Suggestions for Attitudes, Feelings, and Worry

1. I make the time each day to autocondition my mind with a positive attitude.
2. I am happy to be alive.
3. Life is an interesting adventure.
4. I do my best with each situation that arises.
5. I cultivate happiness.
6. As I meet each day, I experience increased confidence, courage, and inner calm that grows with each new experience.
7. Every day I become more perceptive and think more clearly.
8. I fully appreciate myself.
9. I always do what for me is the best possible at the time.
10. I find increasing pleasure and happiness in all that I think and do.
11. I am continually filling myself with humility and strong self-assurance.
12. I find new pleasures in my everyday experiences.
13. I am able to express my delight with my good fortune.
14. I do everything in a relaxed, efficient manner.
15. I listen well and make informed decisions.
16. I have no control over other people, only myself.
17. I am responsible for my thoughts.
18. I am responsible for my feelings.
19. I am responsible for my actions.
20. I do my best to solve the problems I can; I let the others go.
21. I allow others to be responsible for their own thoughts, feelings, and actions.
22. I accept responsibility for my own life.
23. I recognize the difference between "my" problem and "someone else's" problem.
24. I am tolerant, cooperative, and cheerful.
25. By conserving my emotions, I conserve my energy.

Develop a Sense of Humor: It's a Great Tension Reducer!

A healthy portion of laughter can make the daily grind less tedious. It is a mechanism for easing strain. It converts saggy muscles and saddened eyes into a refreshing smile. A humorous attitude may also provide psychological distance from negative images and emotions and may keep you from obsessing on worrisome thoughts. We have all experienced the tremendous feeling of well-being that follows a hearty laugh. We love this quote from Oliver Wendell Holmes:

> The great purpose of life is to live it. Whether my fears are real or imaginary, I will find them less awesome if I strive to participate in the great happenings in the world around me. I am not going to nurse my own fears and unhappiness. If I would have happiness, I must embrace my world, know and learn what makes it "tick." I am going to interest myself in my friends and my family—share their joys and I will be joyful, too.

Happiness, too, is an attitude that can be cultivated. You need not live in constant tension, seldom allowing yourself to smile, and living in an unhappy past. Use self-hypnosis to help you to live in your world today and make yourself responsible for living in it with pleasure.

➠ *Alleviation of Pain with Hypnosis.*   The following case history was taken from the files of the late Dr. William S. Kroger, one of medical hypnotherapy's pioneers.

> Janet, aged 17, had had painful menses since the age of ten. The menses were always irregular. She was forced to retire to bed for 24 to 36 hours after the onset of the pain, which usually occurred about 12 hours after her period began. It consisted of acute lower-abdominal cramps accompanied by considerable nervousness, nausea, and tension. She had received extensive therapy including dilatation and curettage, analgesics, and endocrine preparations.
>
> On August 2, we induced deep hypnosis. Suggestions were given to the effect that her next period would be free from discomfort; that every night before going to sleep she would say to herself, "I will have no pain. I have no dread and anticipation of my next

period." These suggestions under hypnosis were repeated seven times between August 2 and August 29. The period began on September 6, and was remarkably free from pain, although there were slight cramps. Janet did not have to go to bed. After four hypnotic treatments at weekly intervals, using the same suggestions, her next menses, on October 11, was entirely normal in every respect. For one year, without any further treatments, she has been free from pain, nervousness, and all menstrual discomfort. In addition, her periods have been regular.

Hypnosis and Pain Control: It's Nothing New

From the mid-1770s through the turn of this century, hypnosis was a standard medical treatment that seemed to work for people with a variety of medical disorders, primarily relating to pain of some sort or another. However, many doctors stopped using it around 1920 with the advent of psychoanalysis and more sophisticated chemical anesthesia.

Now, nearly 80 years later, the use of suggestion to alter sensory perception, that is, the thought of pain or illness, is becoming an increasingly accepted part of modern medicine. One of the reasons for this is our avid interest in the mind/body connection. As a matter of fact, in 1996, a National Institutes of Health assessment panel recommended that hypnosis and other behavioral therapies be considered medical treatments for chronic pain.

Pain Serves a Purpose

Pain is a brilliant feat of Nature to warn us that something is wrong with our body. It is interpreted in our brains even though the source of the stimulus can be anywhere in our body. It is important to obtain a medical diagnosis to first determine the cause of the pain and to receive any medical treatment recommended for the illness or injury. We do not in any way intend this to take the place of medicine. Self-hypnosis for pain control is meant to supplement, not supplant, medical treatment.

When you know what is wrong, you no longer need the pain. However, you need to keep your brilliant natural alarm system working. You can use self-hypnosis to control any nonuseful pain you have, while maintaining your ability to discern any new problem or change in the current one. If you suffer the pains of illness or injury, the pains of headaches, backaches, arthritis, toothache, or neuralgia, this is good news.

How We "Make It All Better" for Little Children

Think about what we do when we observe a child fall, scrape a knee, and start to cry. Say it's a little boy. As we are cleaning the little one's knee, we may enthusiastically admire the way he was throwing the ball so well and tell him how much we like that baseball hat he's wearing. We may point to his train set and ask him a question about its operation. Like a miracle, the tears stop flowing as he forgets about the pain of his injury and focuses his attention on the train set.

This example points to the critical truth that we've pointed out in previous chapters: We are what we think. We are what we perceive.

Unfortunately, not many of us are capable of simply snapping our fingers and ridding ourselves of what ails us. We need some help, a technique that tunes into our minds and our bodies, too. In order to command the body to behave in a way that is different from the way it habitually behaves requires some new "know-how." Self-hypnosis can help you to gain mastery over physical complaints through the process of distraction, much as we do for little children. Simple, yes, but profoundly effective.

Removing the Feeling of Pain

In self-hypnosis, what we remove is the perception of the pain, or the feeling of the pain. We are filtering out the hurt by shifting our attention away from it. Have you ever had a pain of some kind, such as a headache, and begun watching an exciting movie, only to forget about the pain in your head? That's what will happen when you practice self-hypnosis for pain control. When you have relaxed yourself and are ready to give your subconscious the suggestions, you will just give yourself an alternative "movie" to watch instead of paying attention to the pain. Once again, it's simple, but effective!

We must assume that you have consulted a physician and he or she either has found no physical basis for your complaint or has found an organic source and is treating it. Either way, you are ready to give up the pain. Here is the basis for the technique we offer you in this text: Hypnosis succeeds in relieving your pain by shifting your awareness away from the pain. You have the ability to shift your attention from pain to any other scenario you want to experience.

You can think of your pain as a thing or a color. You can give it a name and a shape. Or you can envision a place you'd love to be. Anywhere is possible, from floating in a hot-air balloon to basking on the beaches of Hawaii. Maybe you'd prefer a scene closer to home or something more "everyday" in nature. Your imagery may relate directly to your afflicted area, but not necessarily. It doesn't matter; the choice is yours. Let your imagination loose and go with it. Remember, the first step is always your autorelaxation. This is essential to self-hypnosis. So, relax yourself completely, and you will be ready to use your powerful mind to reduce your pain.

Some Imagery for Pain Control

- Picture yourself floating on your back in the warm ocean waters off a beautiful Caribbean island. You feel the sun beating down, warming your body, and you feel light and calm as you continue to float.

- Perhaps you've cut your finger or your toe, and it's throbbing. Can your imaging plunge it into a bucket of ice water, so cold that the finger becomes numb?

- Here's an ice image for a headache. Picture yourself setting a large block of ice with a hat-shaped hole in it over your head. It's a perfect fit. You feel some light tingling as the ice cools and numbs your entire head as you sigh, "Ah, that feels good."

- Imagine your pain as a tunnel. You can enter it and exit it. As you enter the tunnel, it is very dark, but as you continue through it, you see a light. As you get closer and closer to the light ahead, your pain becomes less and less intense.

- For a backache: Picture your back as being twice as wide and twice as long as you usually think of it. Imagine all the spaces in your back, lots of spaces for the muscles, nerves, and vertebrae to move around. Imagine the nerves in your back smoothly branching out, no longer gripping and knotting up around each other.

- Think of your pain as a color. When you've chosen the color, decide what shape your pain might be. Then imagine the shape changing, slowly around the sides, first a square, then a rectangle, now perhaps a circle. Just observe the shapes appearing and changing . . . then growing smaller and smaller until you can see only a tiny dot.

- Imagine that you are in a favorite place. Maybe it's a forest setting, or in the mountains. It might be in your own home in a favorite chair. Create in your mind a place that feels safe and secure for you, a place that suggests comfort to your mind. As you see yourself in this place, wherever it is, notice the feelings of relaxation and peace that accompany the picture. Let the peace and comfort begin to flow all through your body. Feel the warmth of the comfort as it spreads to the area of your pain.

- Visualize your pain as a blue mist. See it as a fog of light hazy blue. Take a deep breath, and as you exhale, you can allow the pain to be exhaled into the atmosphere, where it dissipates and disappears.

The Posthypnotic Suggestion Is Important

After you've given yourself the suggestions, it is important that you tell yourself that upon awakening from your trance state, you will feel only at most a slight pressure in the area where you are experiencing pain. You can say to yourself something like, "I may feel pressure or a tingle, even a numbness. Except for that, I will feel light and perfectly comfortable."

Ten Posthypnotic Suggestions for Pain Control

1. I am relaxed and comfortable.
2. I am in control of my body and my responses.
3. I can focus my thoughts on whatever I wish.
4. I find myself feeling better and better with each passing moment.
5. It pleases me to know that I can take a mental trip to anyplace I want to go.
6. Only a slight tingle is present where I once had pain.
7. The slight pressure in my back (or wherever else is hurting) reminds me of my own power to control my thoughts and my body.
8. My life is full of blessings.
9. I approach each day with a positive outlook and a determination to become better.
10. I constantly direct my thoughts toward pleasant things.

A Final Word

Allow us to share with you a quotation from a British colleague, W. J. Ousby, who made an interesting observation that speaks to the divergent roles self-hypnosis has played in pain control. In *Self-Hypnosis and Scientific Self-Suggestions*, he writes, "During recent years, both in Britain and America, soldiers have been trained by using self-hypnotic techniques to render themselves immune from pain and even to undergo torture without betraying military secrets. The self-hypnotic trance is undoubtedly the secret which enables firewalkers and fakirs to perform the feats."

Master Your Emotions Through Self-Hypnosis

Lisa related how, at the age of 12, she discovered a mouse under her pillow. She was frightened and screamed. Her brother had placed it there as a prank, but ever since that episode, she has had nightmares and awakened terrified at the thought of a mouse under her pillow. While in a self-hypnotic state, autoanalysis helped Lisa to trace the source of her unrealistic fear. When she understood the source of her misery, she was able to give herself the autosuggestions to dissipate her fears and get some rest. She repeatedly told herself: I am safe and secure, unafraid and confident. I fall asleep easily, and I sleep soundly and peacefully through the night. I know that childhood pranks are harmless to me now and a child's mischief that happened many years ago has no power over me now. I am relaxed and at peace.

Triumph over Your Fears with Self-Hypnosis

Fear can be classified as one of our most valuable emotions—and one of our most destructive. It can be valuable when it serves the purpose of self-protection and self-preservation. Without being alerted by our fears, we might never survive the many dangers that confront us in life.

Mice, spiders, snakes, fire, heights, thunder, freeways . . . almost everyone is at least a little afraid of something. Unless such a fear is interfering in your life, it is probably well enough just to let it be.

Destructive fears, however, are quite another matter. When they permeate your world and manifest themselves in any debilitating way, however, it is time for you to take control. Fears can lead to something one expert likened to "mental lockjaw." You become afraid to open your mind as well as your mouth. Some fears, programmed into us long ago, can cause us to hesitate and withdraw, or to defensively overreact where forthright, confident action would be more appropriate.

While some of our fears are acquired by abrupt, traumatic experiences, most of our fears are acquired subtly over a period of time. It was the poet Carl Sandburg who wrote, "The fog comes in on little cat feet," and it seems that our fears become a part of us in the same quiet way. They were instilled into us under circumstances where often the intentions were the best. Many children acquire a fear of going to sleep because they have been taught the prayer, "Now I lay me down to sleep . . ." When they come to the part that says, ". . . . If I should die before I wake . . ." they have no desire to go to sleep. Perhaps with all good intentions, they were told when grandmother dies, she's just asleep. It takes only a few suggestions such as these to program a fear into a young child's subconscious mind.

Some children, rightly or wrongly, get the feeling that their playmates might not be approved by their parents, so they refrain from bringing them home. Such a little fear, born in the early years, may well underlie a tendency to be socially unsure in adult life.

Most of your fears were acquired without your fully realizing it. While some of them may have been justified at the time, there may exist no realistic reason for having them now. Yet, because they have been imprinted deep in your memory bank, the subconscious mind keeps yielding them up to your conscious mind for implementation.

It is advisable to examine and periodically appraise fears and emotional reactions. In this process, we come to recognize those fears or feelings that are self-defeating and that should be discarded as inappropriate to our present level of maturity and consciousness. As we explained in the previous chapter, all feelings and emotions can be dissipated when analyzed and the opposite feelings can come in their place.

Is Fear at Fault?

Fear underlies so many of our perplexing emotional states. The following is only a partial list:

Worry is the habit of feeling concerned or fearful.

Guilt is the habit of fearing that you did less than you should, or could.

Loss of self-esteem comes from fear that your conduct falls short of your own ideals.

Loss of self-confidence is born of fear that you will not be able to perform adequately.

Anxiety is an emotional state where habits of fear and hope are alternately present.

Jealousy and envy result from fear or concern that others own or have attained more than you.

Inferiority is a pervasive feeling of fear regarding your own competence and worth.

In addition to being emotionally draining, these negative emotions can make you physically ill. They can erupt into such physical symptoms as headache, high blood pressure, ulcers, nervous disorders, or a compromised immune system. There is even speculation that the formation of cancer cells might be a function of anger-based negative emotions. Many physicians have come forward in the past five years to say that they believe that a patient who has a positive attitude has a higher probability of surviving his or her disease.

Ten General Self-Suggestions for Fear

1. I am relaxed and confident in all situations.
2. I have confidence in my own power to choose.

3. I am prepared and able.

4. I am enough.

5. I forgive myself for past transgressions, looking forward to each new day.

6. I am proud of myself for my accomplishments.

7. I am strong and honest with myself.

8. I practice my self-hypnosis daily, with ever-increasing positive results.

9. I am the master of my responses.

10. I face the future with strength and courage.

Self-Hypnosis Can Help You Conquer Anger

Anger interferes with easy, comfortable living. What we mean by anger is not the brief, often justifiable burst of anger that all of us experience on occasion. That kind of anger is felt, expressed, and forgotten. We mean instead the smoldering, repressed kind that has a different kind of intensity, the kind that results in inappropriate, angry outbursts, temper tantrums, and even physical violence.

Anger is most destructive of all our emotions because it often lies hidden and unrecognized. In *guilt*, we are angry at ourselves. In *hate*, we are angry at the object of our hatred. In *self-pity*, we are angry at the situations or people who frustrate us. Anger may be overt, but often it is insidious in its many disguises. As with other negative emotions, it can be contagious, transmitted from one person to another.

Perhaps you recall being around someone who was ranting and raving about something and being so convincing that you felt yourself becoming angry as well. You may have felt tension building in your neck and shoulders and found yourself clenching your fists, all of this for something that probably had nothing to do with you. The sheer emotion of the anger was pervasive, and it actually contaminated the mood of anyone who got caught up in it.

If you are one who regularly experiences the turmoil of anger or rage, you may be one of those individuals who is thought of as chronically "grumpy"—or a negative person with a "short fuse." Self-hypnosis can help you gain control of your temper and your life.

SELF-HYPNOSIS SUGGESTIONS FOR CONTROLLING A BAD TEMPER

1. I am emotionally mature and responsible.
2. I am capable of making right decisions.
3. I practice and maintain peaceful self-control.
4. I know that I always have the choice to leave any situation.
5. I look for the good in people.
6. I am at peace with myself and with the world.
7. I live happily with other people.
8. I enjoy good physical and emotional health.
9. I like people and genuinely enjoy being around others.
10. I have a kind word and a warm smile for everyone.
11. I know that the key to happiness is love and understanding.
12. I have the ability to smile at those who are angry.
13. I am in control of my emotions.
14. It is easy for me to think clearly and choose the proper words.
15. I am serene and calm.
16. I enjoy being tolerant and forgiving.
17. I am relaxed and comfortable being around others.
18. I cultivate a loving attitude.
19. My subconscious mind guides me to make good, healthful decisions.
20. I accept others as they are.
21. I am experiencing personal growth with each passing day.
22. I surround myself with positive people.
23. I use common sense in my daily life.
24. I enjoy my life.
25. I enjoy regular exercise as an outlet for my energy.

➡ *How Hypnosis Led Joyce to "The Open Road."*   Joyce, who had once been a victim of negative emotions, brought in the following account of her return to "The Open Road."

> In attempting to assemble my thoughts toward expressing what self-hypnosis has done for me, strangely enough, I find myself returning to a poem of Walt Whitman's which I, in younger days and in difficult times, turned to time and again, repeating it to myself, to give me a renewed strength of purpose. The poem is called,
>
> ### THE OPEN ROAD
>
> *Afoot and lighthearted I take to the open road,*
> *Healthy, free, and the world before me,*
> *The long brown path before me*
> *Treading wherever I choose.*
> *Henceforth I ask not good fortune*
> *I myself am good fortune*
> *Strong and content I travel the open road.*
>
> I feel that self-hypnosis has led me again to the open road. I know that the fears, sorrows, apprehensions, and misdirected thoughts were the result of the "weeded growth" of a challenge of which I was not being the master. I learned to look objectively upon my everyday experiences as small and useful building blocks of character.
>
> After I realized this fact, I was able to feel the freedom which pervaded it in all its length and breadth and the challenge that beckoned at its horizon. Self-hypnosis has enabled me to continue my journey and bypass the byroads.

➡ *A Self-Cured Case of Claustrophobia.*   Mrs. Baxter, a woman in her late thirties, described how she was able to conquer her fear of closed spaces (claustrophobia) by means of self-hypnosis.

> I was afraid to get into elevators. Whenever I was caught in a crowd, I felt I would suffocate. I couldn't remain in a room without having to open the door or a window. The thought of being hemmed in threw me into a panic.

After I learned the technique of placing myself in a hypnotic state, I was able to trace my phobia to its root cause. When I was 12 years old, two of my playmates induced me to get into a wooden box. They sat on the lid of the box and wouldn't let me out until I had screamed for help. I thought I was going to die. My mother finally rescued me.

I have given myself repeated suggestions that I can now ride in elevators and found that I was able to do this without feeling panicky. Knowing that I had discovered the cause of my phobia gave me confidence. I realized that my fear of suffocating was nothing more than a carryover from this early unpleasant experience.

I am convinced that tension causes people to be afraid of many things. I practiced the art of autohypnosis by telling myself that I could relax at will simply by thinking about letting my muscles go limp and concentrating on the thought that nothing would happen to me. I was satisfied that I had discovered the cause of my claustrophobia.

At first I would repeat to myself over and over again, "I don't have to fear closed spaces . . . My mind can control my fear of elevators." Now I find that I no longer have to give myself these suggestions. I no longer experience tension and consequently am no longer uneasy or nervous in an elevator.

➠ *A Scientist Overcomes Stage Fright with Self-Hypnosis.* Dr. E., a research scientist in his seventies, had gained an enviable reputation in his field. Because of his outstanding qualifications, he was invited many times to address various audiences, but was inclined to refuse such invitations because he feared he would become too uneasy and nervous. Once, at a convention a year ago, he lectured to a group of scientists and experienced palpitations of the heart, perspiration, and the feeling that he was going to faint.

He realized that fear is an emotion that is influenced by the mind. He knew that if he could learn to control his mind, he would in turn control his fear. He practiced autorelaxation and kept repeating these positive autosuggestions:

I have nothing to fear—I am going to concentrate on the message I wish to pass on to my audience and not on myself—I have confidence in the power of my own mind.

He learned to give himself a session of self-hypnosis before every subsequent lecture and reported that he was able to give many talks afterwards with very little discomfort.

➠ *A Concert Pianist Who Used Self-Hypnosis to Control His Hand Tremor.* A 34-year-old man who had devoted most of his life to the study of music and had given several concert recitals consulted us about a tremor of his right hand, which he had developed within the past year.

Here is his story of what he was able to accomplish with self-hypnosis:

> I was an accomplished pianist and had earned the applause of numerous audiences. During one of my recitals my mind wandered momentarily off to a certain girl I was planning to marry. We had disagreed about our marriage plans. She told me she wasn't quite sure she would go through with the marriage. In the middle of one of my recitals, I experienced a feeling of panic and my right hand began to tremble. Fortunately I managed to complete my concert although I was aware that I had not done my best. I became apprehensive about giving another recital, believing that my hand tremor would reappear.
>
> I memorized the 4-A's method of self-hypnosis.
>
> During self-analysis, I began to solve the conflicts I was experiencing involving my fiancée. For one thing, I was suffering from a fear of being rejected. I had always felt unsure of myself when it came to any relationship with the opposite sex. I came to the conclusion that I was too self-centered. I practiced being more considerate, humble, and less anxious. I developed greater confidence in myself, and my girl finally decided to go through with the marriage. Self-analysis revealed that my tremor had been caused by this frustration.
>
> My final step was to give myself the repeated posthypnotic suggestion that I would be completely relaxed and in full control of

my emotions when playing the piano. I have noticed that I am play-ing better than ever and am happy to say that my hand tremor com-pletely disappeared.

How to Overcome the Fear of Flying with Self-Hypnosis

There are many persons who admit quite frankly that they are afraid to fly. They prefer some other mode of traveling. Some have never been in a plane and attribute their prejudice against air travel to media accounts of airline crashes. They are too scared to take their first trip and are obsessed with the idea that their first experience will be their last. If someone tries to assure them that the odds are in their favor, that considering the many hundreds of thousands of air miles flown without a mishap, they will invariably remind you of some past tragedy that made the headlines. They exclaim: "But, how can you be sure? Every time you step into a plane you are taking a chance. What about unexpected lightning storms? What about mechanical failure? There's no guarantee that you will arrive safely. In a car acci-dent or even a train wreck, you stand some chance of surviving. But when a plane crashes, there are seldom any survivors."

We could go on and on with this kind of negative thinking that people in this group resort to. Some of them have no desire or any intention ever to fly. They feel it is no great handicap if they never get off the ground. But there are those who do have a desire to trav-el by air. They wish they could overcome their fear of flying. They are aware of the many advantages of going someplace by plane. They accept their fear as a decided handicap. They don't know how to go about preparing themselves mentally for their initial flight. They imagine they would panic. The idea of being "shut in—having no place to run to—not being able to get off if they did panic," and so on blocks them from ever going to an airport.

A fear of flying, particularly in today's world, *is* a handicap. We have had the opportunity of helping persons who came to us with this specific problem. We discovered that self-hypnosis proved a most effective method of overcoming their fear of flying.

➠ *The Frightened Flight Attendant.*   In one instance, an airline flight attendant who had survived a crash stated that she had developed a fear of flying and would never fly again. She claimed that her one frightening experience left its mark. She became aware for the first time how "lucky she was," to use her own words. She felt relieved when she gave up her job and was married. Her husband, a businessman, was accustomed to traveling by air and invited her to accompany him on many of his business trips. She refused, admitting that she just couldn't make herself get in a plane again. Since her desire to share his trips was so strong, she decided to try hypnosis and proved to be a good subject.

We introduced her to the technique of abreaction, having her relive and describe under hypnosis the details of her traumatic experience. Following this, she was given the posthypnotic suggestion that she would no longer live in the past, that she would be able to fly again, relaxed and comfortable, and that she would overcome her fear of flying by learning how to apply and practice the 4-A's method of autohypnosis as described in this book.

She has since taken many domestic trips by air and a long-vacation flight to Rome. She reported that she was free of any apprehension and was able to relax and enjoy each experience as she formerly had when she worked for an airline.

➠ *The Two Worried Wives.*   We had two couples consult us who had made plans to fly to Spain for a brief vacation. The husbands had no problem. They had flown many times before. Both their wives were worried, feared the trip, and were acutely apprehensive. Each of them had the experience of going to Florida by plane, but had never crossed the Atlantic. One of them wondered if she should take a strong sedative, thinking it would alleviate her tension. The other was superstitious and feared something would happen because the date of their departure fell on the thirteenth of the month. We instructed them in using self-hypnotic suggestions and assured them that they would find every minute of their experience enjoyable. They did just that.

The reader might feel disappointed if we were merely to say that the way to overcome the fear of flying is to simply practice the technique of hypnotic self-relaxation every day for a week before your prospective trip and all during the time you are in an airplane. Consequently, we are going to give you a few specific things to think about and suggest to yourself; these ideas should be combined with or supplement your autorelaxation and should make it easier for you to achieve the ultimate result you desire:

1. In your day-to-day sessions of autohypnosis suggest to yourself these thoughts: that you *like* airplanes, that you are fascinated by them, that it's a wonderful way to travel, that you are fortunate to be living in an age whereby this mode of travel is available to you, that you are sharing with many thousands of other people the benefits of modern progress. Repeat them to yourself as often as you need to. This develops in you a *positive* attitude about flying. If you *dislike* something and you keep reminding yourself how much you dislike it, it becomes far more difficult to accept or adjust to that which you dislike.

To cite an example, if a person claimed he disliked people, expressed this feeling to others, and kept repeating how much he is bored by people, naturally he is going to feel miserable and have a miserable time at every social gathering he attends. What is he accomplishing by assuming this kind of negative attitude toward people? In fact, he does himself a great deal of harm. As time goes on he takes a *negative* attitude about many other things. We all know people who are predominantly pessimistic, skeptical, and negative. They lose friends quickly because no one wants to be exposed to someone who is "against everything," who predicts the worst and has a gloomy outlook on life.

To overcome your fear of flying, you must develop the attitude that you enjoy and appreciate traveling by air, that it will be an *adventure* for you, a new experience.

2. Condition yourself to the atmosphere of an airport. Watch the planes come and go. Observe the many people buying their tickets, checking their bags, and being met by their friends. Capture the feeling of others. Imagine (via the technique of "visual imagery") that you are arriving by plane. Identify yourself with those you see coming and going. Picture yourself inside a plane. Tell yourself it

must be wonderful to be able to travel, that it's exciting. This kind of positive autoconditioning should prepare you psychologically for your first trip.

3. Take your first trip in a plane with some other person, someone you admire and respect or, better still, with a group of friends who are planning a trip somewhere. This helps you achieve more peace of mind. You begin to console yourself that you are not alone. You begin to think, "If others can travel this way and not feel tense, so can I."

4. Watch the other passengers, including attendants. Remember relaxation is contagious. Let the confidence of the other passengers rub off on you. Make believe you are relaxed. Smile and converse with other passengers. This will help you to get your mind off yourself.

5. Resort to distraction gimmicks. Don't just sit there and worry. Read an interesting book or magazine. Work a crossword puzzle if you like. Whatever it is, keep yourself mentally occupied. It's surprising how quickly time passes, especially if you are having a meal on the plane. Don't give yourself time to think about unfavorable possibilities.

6. Take advantage of the wonderful opportunity you have to practice putting yourself in a state of hypnotic relaxation. Go through the various steps in the early part of the book. Start with muscle relaxation, followed by complete body relaxation, with or without closing your eyes, and then proceed to give yourself some of the preceding suggestions. Talk silently to yourself. Make up your own positive-thinking suggestions.

Here is a sample:

1. I am proud of the fact that I am here on this plane, relaxed and confident.

2. I now relax my body and my mind.

3. I feel fortunate that I am able to get where I am going in such a short period of time.

4. I enjoy my new feeling of self-mastery.

5. I manifest faith in everything I do—faith in the thought that I am secure. My faith in a Higher Power provides me with peace of mind.

6. I make good use of my new habit of hypnotic self-induced relaxation.

7. I now relax each part of my body (progressive relaxation) until my entire body is relaxed (complete relaxation). My body and my mind are relaxed.

8. I am successful in overcoming fears.

These are only sample suggestions, to get you started. As we said before, you can make up your own list and make it as long as you wish. If you follow the guide we have given you, we can almost guarantee you will conquer your fear of flying. You will also be making the conquest of other "unreasonable" fears.

13

You Can Defeat Mental Depression and Unhappy Moods with Self-Hypnosis

Analyze the Nature and Cause of Your Unhappy Moods

Use the following questionnaire in conjunction with the third step of self-hypnosis (autoanalysis). When you are properly relaxed, begin to analyze yourself in relation to your susceptibility to becoming easily depressed.

By studying the answers to these questions, you can find out *why* you become so moody.

	YES	NO
1. Am I too sensitive to criticism?	_____	_____
2. Are my feelings easily hurt whenever I experience the slightest rejection?	_____	_____
3. Do I dislike my physical appearance?	_____	_____
4. Do I get irritable when I'm very tired?	_____	_____
5. Am I shy around people?	_____	_____
6. Do I suffer from indecision?	_____	_____
7. Do I lack self-confidence?	_____	_____

	YES	NO

8. Do I worry about everything? _____ _____

9. Am I living too much in the past? _____ _____

10. Do I feel sorry for myself, seeking sympathy from my family and friends? _____ _____

11. Am I quickly discouraged? _____ _____

12. Am I suspicious of people's motives? _____ _____

13. Do I blame my inadequacies and difficulties on other people? _____ _____

14. Am I too immature to accept ordinary responsibilities? _____ _____

15. Do I seem to be a hypochondriac? _____ _____

16. Do I attribute my depressed moods to some physical condition? _____ _____

17. Am I unhappy and depressed because of resentment, disillusionment, or having been hurt in the past? _____ _____

18. Am I pessimistic about the future?

19. Am I obsessed with the thought that I am a victim of "hard luck"? _____ _____

After you have answered these questions, write down your conclusions. Study them and make the decision that you are going to begin to control these frequent mood swings.

What You Should Know About Mental Depression

There are two general types of depression: (1) normal and (2) clinical. All of us are susceptible to becoming depressed for one reason or another only because we are subjected to both positive and negative influences. If something good happens to us or we succeed in achieving a particular goal, we are naturally happy. On the other hand, if we become greatly disappointed or become chronically ill, we are apt to experience mental depression.

It is important to remind yourself that under certain circumstances *it is normal to become temporarily depressed.* Even psychiatrists who treat depressed patients at times become depressed themselves. All human beings, the poor, the rich, the young, and the old are subject occasionally to unhappy moods.

Many mistaken individuals believe that a normal person is someone who is blessed with good physical health, never gets mentally upset, and maintains a cheerful disposition at all times. So-called "normal" people experience periods of depressions, especially when they meet with a disappointment, but they manage to overcome their unhappy mood.

Note: A deep period of depression that is chronic for more than a few weeks may in fact be a medical problem. In that case, you must seek medical attention. There are many excellent medications on the market today that will ameliorate your depressive symptoms.

However, we have explained that everyday disappointments in life can cause anyone to become depressed. The important thing is how to manage worries and frustrations of everyday life, what our attitude is. If we are hypersensitive to disappointments and frustrations, we seek an outlet through the mechanism of depression and into a dark pool of self-pity.

Some experience states of depression because of some physical handicap or illness. The person, for example, who suffers from an ulcer may be moody and have a sour disposition. It is understandable that someone who is told that he has an incurable disease is likely to be very depressed. One could hardly expect him to feel otherwise. However, psychiatrists know that these unfortunate victims can make their illness more endurable by adopting a peace-of-mind attitude—one of philosophical acceptance.

Any physical condition is capable of influencing the mind and disposition of the individual. Likewise, the mind is also capable of influencing the particular physical ailment. If a patient suffering from a chronic illness allows himself or herself to become more and more depressed to the point of becoming pessimistic about his or her recovery, the chances of being cured are greatly reduced. If, instead, the person were to assume a more hopeful mental attitude, the probability of recovery sooner would be greatly enhanced.

Whether the cause of your depression is a physical illness or an emotional frustration, remember that you always have a choice about your attitude.

Use Posthypnotic Suggestion to Divert Your Mind from Yourself

Our colleague Dr. Henry C. Link told us a story that has a familiar ring to it in the offices of behavioral scientists throughout the country. Laura, a middle-aged patient of his, was complaining of being terribly depressed. She was an intelligent single woman, who had an executive position at a real-estate broker's office. A self-confessed "workaholic," she had, over a period of months, become generally sad and apathetic. Laura knew that her mood was having a detrimental effect on her life, but she was having a hard time just consciously trying to "snap out of it." Laura described how she had begun to dread getting out of bed every morning, not wanting to eat, and generally not caring about her appearance. Her job, which had previously been the center of her life, was suffering as the quality of her work plummeted. Laura had the distinct feeling that if she did not get better, and soon, she would lose her job and everything she had worked so hard to accomplish. Dr. Link began to question her closely, and as he did, it became apparent to him that this woman had a very limited circle of acquaintances and virtually no friends. Although she had worked for many years with some of the other employees in her company, she knew almost nothing about them or their families. She belonged to no groups or organizations outside work, and she didn't even know her neighbors of eight years. At Dr. Link's direction, she started using self-hypnosis, particularly the 4-A's method. One of the things that she focused on in her therapy suggestions was her involvement with other people. The therapy worked wonders for her. She reported to Dr. Link that she was feeling more energetic and alive after the first week. However, the most fascinating outcome of Laura's story was the fact that she had become involved socially with several of her co-workers and their families, and she began volunteering two evenings a week for a local charity for children. At last report, she was so engrossed with her work, her social life, and her charitable efforts that she had no time for melancholy reflections. The moral of this story? Divert your mind away from yourself. Step outside the center of your own being and reach out to someone else. That in itself is great therapy. Coupled with the regular practice of self-hypnosis, it's a fail-safe program to cure depression.

➡ *How Mrs. Lane Conquered Her Depressed Moods with Self-Hypnosis.*   Mrs. Lane, an attractive woman in her middle thirties, had made a habit of negative thinking. She was a confirmed pessimist. Despite the fact that she realized that her *depressed moods* were caused by her dark outlook on life, she experienced a sense of helplessness. She didn't know where to begin or how to bring about a change in her mental attitudes. Her eagerness to learn the techniques of self-hypnosis made her a successful hypnotic subject. She became an entirely "new person" by changing her philosophy of life. Here is her own account of how she thinks *today*:

> I will attempt to describe in the simplest way possible why I choose to make a *positive way of thinking* and *living* a part of my life. Each and every day of my life I plan to live to the fullest by thinking how fortunate I am to be alive. To begin with, I cherish every day I live and can enjoy this wonderful world of ours. I have come to the conclusion that I must think this first and primarily before I can go through each day with pleasant and optimistic thoughts. I don't permit myself to dwell on how difficult or uninteresting a particular job or chore might be. I tackle it and amaze myself that it wasn't nearly as bad as I thought it would be. Time and again I've experienced the feeling that an assignment I simply hated to begin was surprisingly simple once I actually made up my mind to get started and do something about it.
>
> When I feel particularly depressed, I count my blessings right then and there. I say to myself, "What can I complain about and why am I complaining? I am fortunate beyond words. I have health. With this I have a treasure beyond any material thing I could possibly own." I have my health, and with this idea sincerely and genuinely established in my thoughts, I cannot help but begin to feel grateful and

happy. I have instilled in my mind through repeated autosuggestion and self-hypnosis that I have the ability to do whatever I make up my mind to do. As a result I feel not only enlightened but also encouraged because I feel that in just having the gift of good health I have everything. I have come to believe that there are so many lovely amusing incidents that make up our lives. When there is a genuine and sincere interest in everything about you, there is no boredom.

At one time I would awaken in the morning with the thought "What a dreary day I am going to have again—I'm sure everything will go wrong today." Now I realize, "How can anything be pleasant and exciting if I consider it drab and ugly before I have given myself a chance to find out what it will be like—whether I will find it enjoyable or will it suit my taste?" I stifle pessimistic thoughts and instead every morning I start getting myself in the "proper mood" for the day ahead of me. Before getting out of bed, I close my eyes, relax, and concentrate on the idea that this is going to be another interesting day. As long as I think in this fashion, nothing will beat me down. When I have sincerely tried and performed to the best of my ability I experience an inner contentment.

I have personally found that in applying a *positive* approach and a keen, eager interest and determination to reach the goal I set out for without burdening myself with countless pros and cons about whether I can do it, I seldom fail. I try to be myself, enjoy what the other person has to tell me, listen intently, and I cannot help but enjoy whatever I happen to be doing at the moment. In other words, if I am eating an apple, I eat it leisurely and savor the taste. I don't rush to gulp it down, as I had been doing. I take my time and enjoy it to the fullest. I repeat over and over again the suggestion that my life is controlled and regimented by me, and I can choose to make it lovely and happy.

I have learned to channel my thinking to positive thoughts about everything in general, from the most menial tasks to the finest function I may be called on to attend. When I can learn to anticipate a little something in everything I may have to do, or be required to do, amazingly enough it suddenly has some glow and excitement to it, because I thought of it just that way. Life is so beautiful. In conclusion, I have learned this one thing: *As a different person, I now reach out, think happy thoughts, and wonder each day what treasures are in store for me because I dared and tried.*

Twenty Self-Hypnotic Suggestions for Banishing the Blues

Here are some thoughts and suggestions that you can give yourself during self-hypnosis that will help you combat moods of depression:

1. My life is valuable and full of meaning.
2. I have many gifts and talents, and I use them well.
3. I am intelligent, practical, and wise.
4. I really enjoy my own company.
5. I am never alone. I always have my best friend with me—me!
6. I let go of my mistakes and focus on who I am and what I have to do right now.
7. I am grateful for all my blessings.
8. All answers are within me.
9. I give myself permission to be myself. I give myself permission to laugh, giggle, run, dance . . . and cry.
10. I let go of old, outdated ways of behaving, of being.
11. I am a good friend to others and praise others easily.
12. I am fun to be with.
13. I am willing to change.
14. I am growing and evolving all the time.
15. I approach every day with a positive attitude.
16. I move from the old to new ways of thinking and behaving with ease and joy.
17. I am in the flow of life. I move easily through all its currents.
18. I approve of myself.
19. I trust the process of growing and unfolding.
20. I take responsibility for my thoughts, my feelings, and my life.

Chapter 14

How to Create for Yourself a New Personality and a Happier Life

What Is Meant by "Personality"?

Personality is the outward or surface expression of your inner self—
your inner you. It represents a medium of communication. It includes
a combination of many things—the way you walk, dress, eat, and
talk; your tone of voice, facial expression, what you say, how you
say it; your habits—ways of doing things, mannerisms, the way you
express or control your different emotions; your attitude about yourself and others; your desires, dreams, and ambitions; your basic attitude toward life; your likes and dislikes, what you believe and dis-
believe; your ability to love and be loved; your capacity to survive
misfortune. All these things and others constitute your *total you*.
Personality is your *ego, your being*. It is equivalent to the skeletal
framework or structure of your body. When your *ego* collapses,
you are unable to function adequately. Your ego needs constant
support in order to survive. It is responsible for your reaction to your
past experiences, your present mode of living, and your hopes for
the future.

What Made You What You Are

At this moment you are what you are because of a sum total of habit-conditioning influences that helped shape your personality from the day you were born, influences that stemmed from your grandparents and parents, brothers, sisters, relatives, and friends, influences within the home and outside the home, religious influences, the influence of society, the kind of community in which you were brought up (rural or urban), and your many personal past experiences. Just as it takes a variety of colors to make a rainbow, there are many factors that go to make up each personality. No two human beings are exactly alike in everything.

Fortunately, personality traits are not *inherited*. They are expressions of the inner you, which you have *learned* and *acquired* through *conditioning* and *imitation*.

Your personality is influenced by conscious and unconscious factors. Psychoanalysts believe that you can change your personality only by bringing that which is buried in the subconscious mind to the level of conscious awareness. They try to assist you to develop self-insight.

However, with *self-hypnosis* you can accomplish this same thing. Through hypnotic autoanalysis you can uncover the hidden factors in your family background and childhood and evaluate them in terms of their influence on your personality and development. You can resolve guilt complexes that have warped your personality. Using autotherapy (posthypnotic suggestion) you can learn to control your emotions. Mature personality involves self-control. To develop and maintain a healthy personality, you have to work at it consistently by suggesting to yourself during self-hypnotic sessions the personality qualities you wish to acquire. You must begin by changing your attitude toward yourself—you have to stop thinking that you are inadequate. Gradually, a personality shift will occur, deep in the recesses of your subconscious mind. You will notice it when you are conscious of a change in yourself. It will happen in spite of yourself. You will begin to shed your overbearing personality, overcome shyness, become more communicative, or conquer any other specific personality problem you may have.

Can You Change Your Personality?

You can't make yourself taller, but you can develop a *better* personality.

According to Harvard psychologist Gordon Allport, personality involves the interaction of three factors: (1) habits, (2) traits, and (3) attitudes.

A *habit* is something one does over and over again.

A *trait* is a tendency to do something repeatedly in a similar way. For example, a person may have a trait of being untidy.

An *attitude* is a way of looking at something—life, love, relationships.

Habits, traits, and attitudes are *not* inherited. They are learned and acquired. We know that they can be altered. Undesirable habits can be unlearned. You can develop new habits, new traits, and new attitudes using techniques of self-hypnosis. Self-hypnosis can change your appearance, your way of thinking and living.

Many people we know seem not to have changed over the years because they harbor the fallacious idea that you are what you are because of factors in your life that are "fixed." It explains why we often say, "He's a chip off the old block," or "Once a neurotic, always a neurotic."

To change for the better you must be convinced beyond all doubt that you *can* change, that you can learn to become less hostile, antagonistic, and aggressive and overcome emotional handicaps. This conviction must be your starting point in your self-improvement program. It takes recognition of this fact plus determination and application of the principles we are teaching you in this book.

An article in a contemporary magazine related how President John F. Kennedy, in his undergraduate days at Harvard, was a rather introverted, studious young man, whose main ambition in life was to become either a writer or a teacher. He made a dramatic transformation of personality after he decided to enter politics. He made a conscious decision to alter his life direction. Having done that, he overcame his fears and hesitations about public speaking. He developed an extroverted personality that proved a tremendous advantage to him in meeting people and becoming a political success.

You must *want* to change. Many individuals have no incentive to improve themselves only because they were born into a neurotic home and were exposed to the incompatibility of unhappy parents. Or they feel trapped in an unhappy marriage. They take a "What's the use?" attitude. They have self-defeating personalities. You must want to change for your own sake, rather than to please someone else. It is equivalent to keeping clean for your own sake. For example, a woman who becomes fat and blames her obesity on the fact that she is unhappily married might be searching for alibis to excuse her overeating.

Likewise not to improve because you feel it won't be appreciated by someone else is fatal to growth and progress. You reward yourself through accomplishments. You develop a sense of pride, a feeling of worthwhileness and self-satisfaction that enables you to face the future with increasing self-confidence.

No one denies that there is an advantage to having someone encourage you, someone who loves you and has a genuine desire to help you make progress in life. If you have such an advantage it will naturally make it easier for you to attain your individual goals in life. The point we are trying to make is that you do not necessarily need this outside encouragement to bring about self-improvement. No one can stand in your way if you are determined. What you must do is to concentrate on changing and improving yourself every single day.

You will be amazed at the ease with which you effect a transformation of personality and become the kind of person you want to be if you put into practice the suggestions we are about to give you.

The Self-Hypnosis Approach to Personality Change

You can definitely improve your personality with self-hypnosis. You don't have to accept yourself as you are unless you want to. Self-hypnosis can change your inner you for the better. It can help you develop a magnetic personality.

A person with a magnetic personality is one who has developed the ability of holding the listener spellbound, as it were, of captivating an audience, of enchanting a group of people with storytelling. This skill of establishing a quick, favorable rapport with others can be cultivated.

We all prefer to be around people who are relaxed. Relaxation is contagious. We feel uneasy listening to a nervous speaker because of what psychiatrists call "empathy." We *identify* ourselves with someone who manifests self-consciousness, and we become nervous and self-conscious ourselves. On the contrary, the person who is poised and confident makes you feel comfortable. Every time the person laughs, you laugh. This magnetic power of a speaker to put the listener in a hypnotic state, hold the attention of the audience, and convince them of what the speaker is trying to put across is common to successful public speakers. President Franklin Delano Roosevelt possessed this power. His friendly manner of talking during his informal "Fireside Chats" is a good example of this. It has been told that some of the Republican senators didn't trust themselves listening to him because they felt themselves yielding or drawn to his political views.

We know, for example, candidates for public office who had excellent qualifications, yet whenever they addressed the masses they were unable to reach the average person. Though they possessed integrity, sincerity, and other fine qualifications, they had never developed the art of expressing themselves in common, everyday language, of making themselves *loved* by everyone in their manner of talking, facial expression, or other gestures that would tend to emanate humility, confidence, and hope. There are many who are convinced that it was Dwight D. Eisenhower's *popularity* and *likability* that paved his path to the White House. He had been the people's *hero* during World War II. Despite the fact that he was never a senator or a congressman, but a military man, he was still elected overwhelmingly as President of the United States. In a similar way Ronald Reagan, known as "The Great Communicator," had a disarming manner of reaching out person-to-person to people of all political persuasions.

There are numerous examples of others who possess this innate hypnotic or magnetic appeal. It comes naturally to them. It is part of their makeup. The evangelist Billy Graham is apparently endowed with this persuasive power. But we are not all gifted with magnetic personalities. Most of us have to learn and teach ourselves the technique of acquiring personality appeal.

How to Acquire a Magnetic Personality

Start by autosuggesting the idea that you are going to become an *attentive listener*. This invariably flatters the ego of the person talking to you. Try not to interrupt. If you absolutely have to interrupt, preface your remark with "Do you mind if I interrupt for a moment?" Then go ahead and make your point. We all like to feel important. We are all *ego hungry*. We like to be listened to. As you listen, look the person in the eyes. Don't wander off or appear distracted, because it gives the other person the impression that you aren't interested. Your listener may conclude from your wandering gaze that what he or she is saying is not too important to you.

In the motivational classic *The Magic of Thinking Big,* David J. Schwartz makes this interesting observation:

> In hundreds of interviews with people at all levels, I've made this discovery: The bigger the person, the more apt he is to encourage you to talk; the smaller the person, the more apt he is to preach to you.
>
> Big people monopolize the listening.
>
> Small people monopolize the talking.

Let self-hypnosis convert you to becoming a good listener. Resolve that you are going to listen attentively and manifest interest in what the other person is saying by asking an occasional question.

Keep your gaze focused on the person talking to you. This establishes rapport between you and the other person.

An eminent professor of psychiatry was once asked, "What makes a good psychiatrist?" He quickly responded: "One who has learned to become a good listener." Patients like to feel that you are genuinely interested in wanting to hear all about their personal problems.

The same professor was asked, "What other quality makes a good psychiatrist?"—to which he replied, "Make each patient love you." By love, of course, he meant letting the patient develop a respect and confidence in your integrity. He added, "Become sympathetic. If you must be firm, be kind. Don't scold. Educate instead. Don't tell a patient about the stupidity of his past mistakes. Tell him what you think he is capable of accomplishing. Inspire hope. Conveying the impression that you are condemning him for his wrongs is only adding to his frustrations. A patient comes to you to be encouraged, not to be admonished."

Psychoanalysts use the term "positive transference" to refer to the establishment of a favorable rapport with their patients. A good doctor-patient relationship is essential to a patient's recovery.

A good interpersonal relationship between you and another individual or a group is also essential to your success in life. You have to make a conscious effort to make other people believe in you, believe in what you think and say.

Give yourself the posthypnotic suggestion that you are going to think before you speak, being careful not to offend anyone, that you are going to give people the feeling that you are a sincere and warm person. Practice being simple in your language so that you are understood. After all, speech is a form of communication. If very few people understand what you're driving at, your efforts will prove futile. It is equivalent to receiving a letter from someone whose handwriting is so illegible that you can't make it out.

Ten Posthypnotic Suggestions to Give Yourself for Getting Along with Others

1. As I meet and deal with other people, I remember to practice being relaxed and friendly.
2. I listen attentively when someone else is speaking to me, keeping my eyes on the speaker's.
3. I strive to put others at ease by my outgoing, sincere manner.
4. When I am with the opposite sex, I am comfortable and relaxed.

5. I seek ways to make others feel good about themselves.

6. My confidence grows every day.

7. My social skills improve every day.

8. In times of stress or confrontation, I remain inwardly calm and secure.

9. I take time to understand others' perspective.

10. I always have a choice.

Develop a Tolerant Personality with Self-Hypnosis

Remind yourself that the world does not belong to any one race. The stars, the oceans, the moon, the mountains, and the rivers belong to no one. Everything we acquire, we leave behind. It is also important to remind yourself to be humble. If a photographer were to intermingle the adult population of the world and have every human being stand elbow to elbow for a single group picture (assuming that it could be done), can you imagine how long it would take for people, whether they were kings or queens, millionaires or truck drivers, to find themselves in a rolled-up photograph of a veritable sea of human beings? This should give you some idea of how insignificant we really are. When we speak of the world in terms of millions of years, you can appreciate how it compares to the average span of humankind's life—our few years of life are only a grain of sand on the beach of life. It takes this kind of reality and humility to appreciate, *tolerate*, and respect the rights of *all* people as human beings. Progress cannot exist without successful interpersonal relationships. Our world should be one of sharing—a sharing of material things as well as ideals.

The point of it all is that you must assume a proper attitude about people in general before you can learn self-hypnotic techniques for getting along with the people you come in contact with. To become *tolerant* of people you must love life—you must like yourself and your surrounding world.

During a self-hypnotic session, suggest the idea that tolerance is one of the major personality assets that you want to acquire. Tell yourself that people will get under your skin, to use a common expression, only if you let them. Anyone can get along with a mature individual. The real challenge and test of maturity is to learn to get along with people who are difficult and unhappy. Everyone has to deal with hard-to-get-along-with people, whether they like it or not.

A role to follow and one to include under autosuggestion is to repeat each day, "I respond to all people in a reasonable, relaxed way."

Enlist the Cooperation of Your Friends for Personality Improvement

Let your friends know that you are trying to improve your personality. Ask them to be frank with you. Have them give you some honest, constructive criticism. After all, they have had the opportunity of observing you. Assure them beforehand that you are not going to be oversensitive and resent their honest evaluation of you. You can learn much about yourself by enlisting the opinions and advice of your friends. Ask them for suggestions as to what they think you can do to improve yourself. In the long run, they will admire and respect you for your willingness to change.

In doing this, be prepared to *accept* whatever advice you are given that you regard as constructive.

➠ *Alice Acquires a New Personality Through Self-Hypnosis.* Alice had been an introvert practically all of her life. Her parents died when she was a child. Brought up by an aunt who was strict, she developed a deep sense of inferiority early in life. Her aunt made all her decisions for her. As a consequence, when she grew up she manifested a complete lack of confidence. Although she managed to support herself as a typist-clerk, Alice never achieved enough maturity to establish a normal adjustment to the opposite sex or to people in general. She attributed this gap in her life to extreme shyness. She refused social invitations because she was too self-conscious to participate in a friendly conversation with anyone.

Even at church functions she seldom spoke to someone else she knew. She was aware of the fact that her loneliness in life was caused by her own refusal to make friends. When Alice could no longer "go on," to use her own words, when she was getting more and more "depressed," she decided to seek help. She had been wallowing in self-pity.

Alice was taught the techniques of self-hypnosis as outlined in Chapter 5. She began using it around people. She also learned how to use self-suggestion to her advantage. She told herself, after being able to induce her own hypnotic state, that she was becoming more communicative. She practiced smiling more and made herself go out more to the theater, to someone's home, to a concert. By doing more talking and becoming more friendly, she gradually began to come out of her shell.

Self-hypnosis enabled her to make plans. She told herself she would take a trip to Europe, which became a reality. Her friends told her about the remarkable change in her personality. She told them that she finally awakened to the realization that she had the capacity to overcome her shyness—that through self-hypnosis she was able to develop a feeling of self-confidence. Even her voice changed. At one time it was weak and childlike in quality. Now she spoke in a more assertive manner. She learned to gesticulate and vary her tone of voice and observed that she was able to hold her listener's attention. She looked different because she felt different inside. Alice claimed she could always rely on a session or two of self-hypnosis to carry her through any trying or challenging situation. She takes pride in having developed an extroverted type of personality and is no longer handicapped by her shyness.

Here are some of the things we taught Alice to repeat to herself during her self-hypnosis sessions:

1. I practice my self-hypnosis skills every day. As I do, relaxation becomes easier and easier for me.

2. I am overcoming tension and replacing it with calmness.

3. I am becoming more confident, self-assured, and courageous every day.

4. I know that all the power I need is within me.

5. I work hard to be a productive, useful human being.

6. I release all feelings of self-consciousness and replace them with self-love.

7. I offer myself in constructive service to others.

8. I get along easily with other people. I am warm and friendly.

9. I am poised and in control of my responses.

10. I always have a choice.

Self-Hypnosis Improves Your Memory and Ability to Learn

Ralph Daigh, a writer, reports how a young man in his final year of medical school at an eastern university told him how he had been using self-hypnosis throughout his undergraduate and postgraduate days, for the most part with the full knowledge of his professors. Daigh informs us that he made Phi Beta Kappa, had the highest grades in his class at medical school, and was offered possibly the highest salary ever offered an intern to stay at the school's hospital for several years of hypnotic research. This young man, so Daigh tells us, is the son of a professional hypnotist, and his grandfather was both a physician and a hypnotist.

There are many theories about learning, ranging from complex formulas to Plato's simple assertion that learning is simply discovering what we already know. It is not necessary, however, to understand anybody's theory of learning to be a better learner. We've found that it is most often a case of developing better study habits and improving your memory.

The ill effects of poor study habits are not confined to the classroom. If you have an exam, a progress report, a sales presentation—any act that requires preparation of new material—you can turn it into a dramatic, punishing experience by delaying your study. On the other hand, the simple act of managing your time makes it a completely different scenario. Self-hypnosis makes time management a reasonable goal.

As for memory, remember the earlier data in Chapter 3 about the storage capacity of your brain. In your lifetime, you will store billions of bits of information. For example, it has been estimated that the word-storage bank of the average person contains some 50,000 words. Some come to mind immediately; others must be searched for, but they are all there. Once learned, the material can be brought forth. That is where self-hypnosis can be of infinite value.

Fifteen Self-Suggestions for Learning and Memory Improvement

1. When I have something to learn or prepare, I begin by planning my time wisely.
2. I have a specific time set aside each day with goals to accomplish toward my study.
3. I am diligent in my study habits.
4. I am confident in my time-management ability.
5. I make sure I have all the resources I need at my side at each study period.
6. I begin my study by relaxing myself completely.
7. My powers of concentration are sharp and focused.
8. My retention of the new material is strong and certain.
9. I approach new learning situations with enthusiasm.
10. My positive attitude serves me well in my study. I know I can do it.
11. I am a self-disciplined person.
12. I am prepared.
13. I have all of the power of my subconscious mind at my disposal.
14. I recall what I know with ease.
15. I always have a choice.

Self-Hypnosis for Concentration and Study

The ability to concentrate is something you can *develop* and culti-vate—something you can *learn*. Many of us handicap ourselves by harboring the fallacy that we simply are unable to concentrate. We believe, erroneously of course, that our difficulty in concentrating is due to something we cannot explain. We rationalize and tell our-selves that some people are just naturally gifted that way as if they were endowed at birth with special powers of concentration.

You have been taught that self-hypnosis is a technique, a psy-chological tool for achieving self-discipline, self-relaxation, and self-improvement. This is accomplished by means of self-suggestion during the trance or hypnotic state, the state of complete relax-ation. If you wish to increase your powers of concentration, repeat the following self-directed suggestions during your sessions of self-hypnosis:

1. I can concentrate.
2. I make concentration a *habit.*
3. I reduce distractions to a minimum whenever I am reading or studying.
4. I am an intelligent person.
5. I easily achieve my goals.

➠ *How Self-Hypnosis Enabled Norman to Become a Better Student.*   Here is Norman's own account of what he was able to accomplish with self-hypnosis.

> My grades in school were poor because I was unable to concen-trate. I was constantly looking off into space and daydreaming about one thing or another. I worried about my grades.
>
> I told Mr. Berger about my problem, and he recommended that I try hypnosis.
>
> I learned how to relax and practiced what I had been taught. For example, I would make myself comfortable by removing my shoes and loosening the top buttons of my shirt. I then let myself go limp. I told myself I could feel the muscles of my eyes getting tired

and that I would soon close my eyes. I felt the relaxation travel from my eyes down my arms and legs until I felt completely relaxed. I told myself that I would also relax my mind as well as my body. I made myself think of something pleasant and remained in this state for 15 to 30 minutes. I then gave myself the suggestion that I would con- centrate better and improve my study habits. I counted to ten and opened my eyes suggesting that I would feel confident and would overcome my fear of taking tests, that I would be able to remember what I had studied and would get better grades. I gave myself this suggestion daily for many weeks.

My grades have improved, probably because I am able to relax for the first time before and during examinations. When I am relaxed I find that I am better able to think. I have also used hypno- sis to help me with other problems.

⟫ *Self-Hypnosis Changed Barbara's Life—Helped Her Achieve Greater Success.* While we appreciate Barbara's flattering indebt- edness to us for helping her achieve success as an author, we feel she is the one who should be congratulated, for it was her own deter- mination and faith in self-hypnosis that accounted for her "dream success" becoming a happy reality.

Barbara had always wanted to write a book. She "dreamed" about it. However she found herself "mentally blocked," as she put it, whenever she made an attempt to get started.

Despite the fact that she had experience as a newspaper reporter, she was unable to convince herself that she had the ability to write her first book.

After mastering the techniques of self-hypnosis, as described in Chapter 5, she began noticing that she was able to put her thoughts on paper more readily and soon discovered that she had managed to complete a final draft of her book.

We asked her to jot down some of the things she suggested to herself and how she achieved what she had.

I learned to overcome the greatest hurdle of all—sitting down at the computer. I could think of a million reasons why I wasn't ready at the moment to start working.

Using the 4-A's method of self-hypnosis, I taught myself to relax. I told myself I was going to discipline myself by awakening at 6:00 every morning and writing for two hours before I did another thing. It soon became a habit. I used self-hypnosis to inspire confidence in myself. Before long, I realized that I had achieved my goal. I had the satisfaction of having written my first book.

It has been many years since Barbara came to us, wanting to know how she could use self-hypnosis to attain her one big wish in life.

We are happy to report that Barbara has had two books published, one of which was purchased by a Hollywood producer and made into a movie. In one of her letters she wrote:

A wonderful side result of the book writing is that I now write feature articles and stories instead of straight news and consequently earn more than I did previously at my regular newspaper job. Self-hypnosis has changed my life!

How to Achieve Hypnotic Power for Yourself and Influence over Others

Repeat during self-hypnosis: Others automatically respond to me in a more positive way because

1. I am kind and unselfish.
2. I am willing to do favors when I can.
3. I smile more.
4. I listen well.
5. I make conversation interesting.
6. I avoid sarcasm.
7. I exercise tolerance.
8. I control my emotions.
9. I am courteous and polite.
10. I am sincere and try to be myself.
11. I think before I speak.
12. I avoid being overcritical.
13. I try to understand why people behave as they do.
14. I act friendly and cheerful.
15. I compliment people for the things that deserve praising.

16. I appreciate people.
17. I make other people feel important.
18. I mind my own business.
19. I am a positive person.
20. I radiate enthusiasm.

What Getting Along with People by Using Self-Hypnosis Can Do for You

1. *Bring you greater success in your job or career.* According to Lee Giblin, author of the book *How to Have Confidence and Power in Dealing with People*, "The Carnegie Institute of Technology analyzed the records of 10,000 persons and arrived at the conclusion that 15 percent of success is due to technical training, to brains and skills on the job, and 85 percent of success is due to personality factors in the ability to deal with people successfully."

He also informs us, "When the Bureau of Vocations Guidance at Harvard University made a study of thousands of men and women who had been fired they found that for every one person who lost his or her job for failure to do the work, two persons lost their jobs for failure to deal successfully with people."

Giblin concludes that 66 percent of all failures in the business world are failures in human relations—that so-called personality problems, such as timidity, shyness, and self-consciousness are basically problems in dealing with people.

2. *Provide opportunities for other people to help you.* An executive or boss is most likely to help someone who is likeable. When you make friends easily, you become popular. Persons who are popular are usually extroverts. They are entertaining. They like to make other people happy. They enjoy life more, and as a result of making numerous friends, they capitalize on their contacts to advance themselves. They know that it doesn't pay to be shy, that it is normal to ask favors and to know what you want out of life. More people are willing to help you than you realize if you just ask for their help.

3. *Give yourself opportunities to help others.* Happiness in part comes to you when you make other people happy. People like you if you show them that you are unselfish. Happiness includes giving, receiving, and sharing. We are all dependent on one another for happiness. You can make people happy. They can make you happy. If you make it your business to get along with people, you will experience an inner contentment, self-satisfaction, and a feeling of accomplishment. Look for ways of helping others—they can be found.

4. *Increase your self-confidence and self-esteem.* If you know others like you, you are bound to be proud of yourself. You become less shy. You get to like making new friends. You begin to develop the techniques of feeling at ease in the presence of others and of putting others at ease. You are no longer frightened by people. You discover that the secret of making friends is to act friendly and cheerful. People will accept you if you're sincere and manifest a genuine wish to be a friend.

Self-Hypnosis Enhances Sales Ability

Manufacturers have long recognized the tremendous value in publicizing and advertising their products. The public is influenced by the cleverness and attractiveness of advertisements. As we have said many times in this book, our minds are influenced by what we think, what we hear, and what we see. You have often heard someone say, "I couldn't resist buying it." It's not always the product that counts; it's how it's described and promoted. *Hypnotic appeal* plays an important role in the field of selling and advertising. People must be made to *want* to buy a particular product. Publishers are aware of this. The mail-order catalog must be so worded that the individual is made to feel that he or she *needs* the item that is being advertised, that it will have tremendous value for him or her, and that he or she will benefit in many ways from the product. That's why titles of books are so important. They must be provocative. The reader's curiosity must be aroused. Paperback covers try to quickly capture your attention, via sensational titles and compelling pictures. This "visual appeal" we have talked about comes under the category of "hypnotic equivalents."

People who are successful in sales are adept at using hypnotic principles, although most of them don't realize it. They know that the first thing they must sell is themselves. Some people seem to have the intuitive ability to gain rapport, and they are invariably the ones who make the most successful salespeople. A winning personality, a positive attitude, and a sincere desire to help are all traits that, when combined with a knowledge of the product or service, make the sale every time.

The characteristics of sales success can be learned. The same principles apply whether you are selling cars, real estate, magazine subscriptions, insurance, or computers. Personality appeal is really hypnotic appeal. The persuasive personality of an excellent salesperson comes from a sense of self-confidence and general knowledge of what he or she is selling. Such a person is focused and organized with a plan for each day. As with any other area of your life you want to improve, you must make a list of self-given suggestions to use each day in your self-hypnosis practice. You will make your own personalized list, of course, but we will give you a few here to get you started:

1. I wake up every morning with the expectation of having a good day.

2. I experience a feeling of inner confidence and peace as I plan my day.

3. I am completely familiar with the product or service I am selling.

4. I believe in the value of what I am selling, and I am proud of my job.

5. I am careful in my grooming so that I make an excellent first impression.

6. I listen to my customers so that I may be able to better meet their needs.

7. I study my sales prospects so that I may tailor my responses to them more appropriately.

8. I give sincere and well-meaning compliments to others when it is justified.

9. I am continually seeking self-improvement through education and observation.

10. I always have a choice.

Visual Reminders

We believe in recommending *supplementary* methods of achieving self-improvement goals. Giving yourself messages by printing something on a note paper and tacking it on a wall in your room may help you stick to a given resolution. It provides a constant suggestion for your subconscious to absorb. Everyone can make use of this system. On the highways you come across signs such as "Stay Alive—Keep Awake" or "Drive Safely—Live Longer." The sign "Think" actually makes people cautious around dangerous machinery. They are less apt to do something carelessly. If you are tense and nervous, perhaps it might be well to put a "Relax" sign where you can see it every day. It's not what we know, it's what we forget to do. We need constant reminders. Everyone knows it's better to be calm and relaxed, but how many of us remember not to get emotionally upset? As businesspeople, teachers, husbands, wives, and parents, we forget, and before we realize it we're in some sort of emotional outburst.

Let's face it. Our minds are influenced by thousands of suggestions in something we see—a sign or a picture. Why not capitalize on this naturally occurring tendency? We are all receptive and susceptible to "visual suggestions."

If you want to lose weight, find some old pictures of yourself when you were slender, have them enlarged, and look at them every morning and night. It will serve as an incentive for you to reduce. It will be a daily reminder.

If you lose your temper at the drop of a hat, print a sign "Keep Calm" and stick it up where you can see it all day long.

It sounds childish, but what's the difference if it works? When you've achieved what you're after, you no longer have to put up signs to look at. You will have developed by then the *habit* of keeping calm.

You sometimes see signs such as "Smile" in restaurants. It's surprising what effect this has on both the waitress and the customer. It all comes under the category of "Visual Suggestive Therapy."

Twenty Self-Suggestions for Increasing Your Hypnotic Power and Appeal

1. I genuinely like other people.
2. I give generously to myself, and I give generously of myself to others.
3. I am enjoyable to be around.
4. I see the good in others, and I seek to bring it out.
5. I bring a positive attitude to everything I do.
6. I respect myself.
7. I practice tolerance and respect for others.
8. I release prior resentments and move on.
9. I have a variety of interests in life.
10. My goals are high, and I reach them easily.
11. I do things as they need to be done.
12. I treat others as though they were what they want to be.
13. I am honest with myself and everyone else.
14. I easily show warmth and concern for others.
15. I quietly do worthwhile things for others.
16. I praise others freely and sincerely.
17. I am patient with those who see things differently from the way I do.
18. I am prepared.
19. I radiate strength of purpose.
20. I always have a choice.

Chapter 16

Using Hypnotic Magic to Stay Young and Live Longer

You Are As Old As You Feel

To expect self-hypnosis to be successful in helping you to stay young longer and enjoy happier living, there are many things you must know about the problem of growing old gracefully.

For one thing, you should convince yourself that there exists a great deal of literal truth in the proverbial expression, "You are as old as you feel."

Dr. Wilhelm Stekel, one of the original collaborators with Professor Sigmund Freud in the field of psychoanalysis, wrote that age is a relative factor—that some men of 30 feel like men of 60, and vice versa, men in the calendar age of 60 not uncommonly feel as though they are still in their thirties. He concluded there was only one true means of rejuvenation: keeping your heart everlastingly young, being able to burn spiritually for ideals, for all that is beautiful in this world and for all that can thrill you emotionally.

Make Happier Living Your Goal

No one wants to prolong life for the mere attainment of old age. We want to live longer only if we can make the harvest years of our life both healthful and enjoyable. We want to know how we can keep young in spirit.

One of the first requirements for achieving successful results with self-hypnosis insofar as growing old gracefully is concerned is to accept the self-given suggestion, "I am not necessarily as old as my arteries, but rather I am as old as I feel." This should be your key formula for staying young.

By achieving serenity of mind through techniques of self-hypnosis, you will be adding years to your life. In previous chapters we gave you specific suggestions as to how you can conquer fear, eliminate tension, and master the art of relaxation. This in itself will aid you in experiencing peace of mind during your entire life.

If you have learned to use self-hypnosis to improve your living habits and to give you better health, then you can expect to add a number of years—possibly an extra decade—to your normal life expectancy. But as we pointed out, your goal should be not to merely live longer, but to have a richer, happier life.

A Theory of Aging: Mind over Body

There are many theories and explanations as to why we grow old, why some of us grow old prematurely, why others develop symptoms of senile thinking. There are those who never seem to grow old, while some decrease their span of life by having lost their will to live.

Personally, we are inclined to the opinion that aging is due to a deficiency in the quantity and quality of *succus de vitae*, to coin a phrase, which means "juice of life"—a combination of hormones and secretions of all our endocrine glands. It is our own theory of the mind/body relationship.

Scientifically, no one can deny the dynamic influence that these secretions have upon our minds in the production of complex emotions. Mind and body can no longer be considered as divorced entities. From the moment we draw our first breath, we begin to express our feelings through various behavior reactions as a body-soul unit, from crying, fretting, nail biting, thumb sucking, temper tantrums in childhood to impulsive decisions, elations, and depressions of adolescence.

The emotional tone or the so-called "affectivity" of an individual is closely associated with the vital functions of the visceral organs. The famous surgeon Dr. George Washington Crile once said that "When stocks go down, diabetes goes up." Have you ever appreciated the effect a quarrel or a bad-news phone call may have on your appetite? How worry is able to drag down the normal weight of an individual? How recovery from a critical illness results in a renewed determination to live?

Every doctor can relate many instances where this will to live has perhaps the deciding factor in the recovery of a patient.

It is this very phenomenon of the influence of the mind over our body organs that also influences our longevity. Negative thinking can curtail your life span.

➡ *Through Self-Hypnosis, Henry Discovered One of the Secrets of Longevity.* Henry informed us that a few years ago he experienced what he described as the greatest frustration of his life—his greatest sorrow. His wife died of cancer at the age of 57.

Here is the story of Henry and his tragic misfortune and how self-hypnosis helped him develop a new philosophy of life.

Henry had planned to retire to Florida after 30 years of married life. He and his wife made extensive preparations for the building of their dream house, where they would spend their remaining years in comfort. Henry's wife was an accomplished artist, and she planned to devote full time to painting. Henry, on the other hand, a retired engineer, took courses in woodworking. He made this his hobby and thought he would find enjoyment and serenity in making frames for his wife's paintings, plus other woodworking activities. He longed to do something with his hands, to compensate for the many years he devoted to mental or "brain-work," as he put it.

He looked forward to living out his life in a warm climate, in a beautiful home, equipped with a studio for his wife and a workshop for himself.

But fate struck a cruel blow. His wife was stricken with a gall-bladder attack and within three months succumbed to cancer. Henry's world had come to an end. He died emotionally. Nothing was of interest to him. When we met him, he had become 20 years older than his calendar years. Henry became depressed, lonely and had lost his will to live. His sister, who was deeply concerned about him, suggested that he consult a psychiatrist.

Following several interview consultations, he consented to learn how he might help himself with techniques of self-hypnosis. We acquainted him with such terms as autorelaxation, autoanalysis, and autotherapy. We explained how self-hypnosis works and what he had to do to make self-hypnosis successful.

At this point, we would like him to describe in his own words the results he obtained:

> I kept repeating to myself, using the method of hypnotic self-suggestions, that I had much to live for, that I had to carry on in memory of my beloved wife (for that is the way she would have wanted it), to continue discharging responsibilities to my children. Self-analysis, self-relaxation, self-hypnosis were terms that seemed meaningless to me, but patiently and with understanding these powerful aids were explained to me. During the sessions that followed, I gradually began to dispel my feelings of self-pity and finally concluded that to succumb to grief was abnormal and fruitless. While I realized that the source of my former happiness could not be regained, I could at least, by changing my attitude, seek peace of mind. I thereby resolved to make myself useful, to offer a hand to others who seemed in more desperate need of help. A more cheerful pattern on my part succeeded in overcoming irritable selfish tendencies and anxieties that were insidiously manifesting themselves. I began to find satisfaction in doing odd repair jobs for my friends, in helping children with their schoolwork, in vocational guidance, in giving talks on some of the latest achievements, and in making useful to others through some of the knowledge gained in almost four decades of speciality in my profession. I began to read books I wanted so much to read, but for which it seemed I could never find the time. I found enjoyment in listening to good music, in watching television, and in more closely following world developments. I would save the editorial section of the Sunday papers so that I could peruse the news more intelligently during the week. I would clip poetry and illustrations that I knew would have pleased my wife. Her paintings in my room became a source of inspiration to me and

afforded the required courage to carry on. I decided to go to Europe with my sister, and there I saw the places and people I wanted to see. Gradually I was acquiring a changed and healthy attitude of life. I was becoming younger instead of older. I had not realized that the right outlook could overcome my misfortune. I told myself repeatedly that I *could* survive this great disappointment in my life.

After a long period of adjustment through self-hypnosis and self-analysis, I began to see rays of hope, and life had meaning again. I had learned to live alone; I was making new friends. No longer did I dread solitude and old age. I was accepting my destiny without complaint. When periods of depression arose, I would seek relief in self-hypnosis. I would think of my children and grandchildren, how happy they were to see me coming to their homes. I would think of the happy days spent in Boy Scout activities where I observed the eagerness of youth in the pursuit of knowledge and of service to others. In brief, I replaced *negative* thinking with *positive* and *optimistic* thoughts. I would not allow myself to fall again a victim of self-pity. I truly began to relax and take things in their stride as they occurred each day. I was finding peace with myself at last. Utilizing the power of self-hypnosis enabled me to adjust myself intelligently, unemotionally, and healthfully to what I had feared was my greatest life's frustration. I overcame my sorrow with repeated suggestions that I could live out my remaining years fruitfully by helping others and by maintaining my faith in the goodness of other people in the world. I am also planning on remarrying.

I am confident that as long as I can continue to enjoy this peace, as long as I remind myself of the saving power of the human mind, I shall never grow old in the true sense of the word.

Let Your Work Become Your Hobby

Many people are bored with life because life is drudgery to them. They remind themselves how much they dislike their work, how they hate going to work, and how tired they are after eight hours at their job. These same people complain even when they change their job. Nothing ever seems to satisfy them. Many of them are chronic complainers. They are victims of a negative attitude about everything. But this can be changed. Self-hypnosis is a technique for changing yourself by changing your attitude. Once you accomplish this, all life takes on a different perspective. You begin to feel healthier, happier, and less tired.

Here is some excellent advice from Dr. Alfred J. Cantor, a physician-author, who substantiates from his own experience what we have just said.

> Simplify life by letting your work become your hobby. Learn to like what you do to the point where you look upon it as a hobby. Again, it is merely a matter of attitude. As a physician, I see a great many patients. Many of these patients ask me why I work so hard, or how I keep up the pace.
>
> The answer is very simple: "I never work. I enjoy what I do." You see—it is a matter of attitude.
>
> If you have the proper attitude, you can be active practically 20 hours a day with only four hours' sleep—and yet honestly say that you "never work." You must learn to enjoy what you do to such an extent that you are happiest when you are busy. But you are not at work.
>
> When you have achieved this goal at the end of a very busy day, you will be full of energy, raring to go. Otherwise, you may work a six- or eight-hour day—doing something you don't enjoy—and be extremely tired and ready only for bed at the end of that short day.

If boredom and fatigue are interrelated, why allow yourself to become bored? Enthusiasm dispels boredom. Enthusiasm is something that can be developed through self-hypnosis, or more specifically through the technique of self-suggestion. The *right attitude* toward everything you do makes everything a lot easier.

Hypnosis and Religion

We read in the newspaper about a Methodist pastor in Georgia who has been using hypnosis to help his subjects in solving problems. He has found it a helpful aid in counseling some 200 persons. The pastor states that he "often has been able during the past two years to penetrate a "wall of resistance" that prevents many individuals from responding to everyday counseling techniques.

By bypassing the conscious mind in difficult cases, the minister not only gets at the seat of problems more directly, but also can help to achieve more effective solutions.

Self-Hypnosis Makes Prayer More Effective

The late Dr. William J. Bryan wrote an excellent book entitled *Religious Aspects of Hypnosis*. In it, Dr. Bryan attempted to show how prayer is akin to a state of hypnosis and how the prophets produced visions by hypnosis: "Prayer is a state of mind, an altered state of consciousness, a specific kind of hypnosis. The conversation of prayer is merely the communication between the mortal and his God."

As to whether our prayers are answered, Dr. Bryan wrote:

The fact that millions of individuals actually receive what they pray for supports the idea that if what one prays for is genuinely good for him, and if the prayer in itself is in earnest and properly executed, it will, quite amazingly be frequently answered in the affirmative.

He added:

In order to receive the affirmative answer to one's prayer it is important to *believe*. This can only be accomplished when it is done on a level of deep emotion within the recesses of the deepest parts of our mind and soul. This "sincere true belief" is only felt by the employment of hypnosis.

The prophets produced their visions by a form of autohypnosis, and in the Middle Ages most of the prophets who heard the voice of God actually dissociated their own voices and heard themselves. The visions of Ezekiel and Daniel were definitely produced by autohypnosis and men were shown in dreams what was suggested to them by their own thoughts.

In another section of his book Dr. Bryan pointed out:

> Many theologians of that era used auto-hypnosis to deepen their
> own religious experience enabling them to remain closer to
> their own personal Gods. Many elements of hypnosis remain in
> our religion today. The chanting, testimonials, the flickering can-
> dles and the cross as a fixation point for our vision; the relax-
> ation of the rest of our body; the bowing of our heads in sup-
> plication; the silence in the Friend's meeting; cabala in Jewish
> mysticism; the Preparation for prayer; the rotation of the body
> in the synagogue, and the effect of prayer on those who offer it
> are all examples of hypnotic techniques which have been
> accepted as part of our own religious experience.

We are very pleased to know that there are those who recognize the value of what we might call the "hypnotic approach." A
clergyman needs to develop a hypnotic personality—radiating positive rapport with his parishioners. He must give them a feeling of
comfort, a feeling of relaxation, a feeling of confidence. The *new
approach* has no place for shouting, threatening sermons. People
are seeking peace of mind. They don't want to be frightened and
made to feel guilty. The voice of the pastor must be soothing as the
organ music. His Sunday message must bring comfort and hope to
those in need of spiritual encouragement. More people would attend
church regularly if clergymen would use their hypnotic powers to
dispel people's fears and superstitions. Instilling the fear of hell for
the punishment of our sins is a *negative* approach.

Autohypnosis recognizes the existence of God-Power in all of
us. It is allied to mind-power, a force for good. It enables us to overcome fear, to survive personal misfortunes, and to inspire courage
in others. God-Power is a self-healing power.

Self-hypnosis should help you supplement your weekend
church religion with an *inner religion*, a seven-day-a-week religion—
a religion of *love without fear*—a religion of *positive thinking*.

Prayer becomes more effective when self-hypnotic techniques
are employed. The person who has achieved self-mastery through
self-hypnosis is better able to experience inner peace, because he or
she believes and has faith in the power of love that exists within
him.

Autohypnosis and church religions have common goals—self-improvement, via positive suggestions, self-forgiveness, love of our fellow human beings, faith in humankind, and a belief in a Higher Power, a Divine Power that is omnipotent.

Self-hypnosis can make you more amenable to the help you seek from your particular church religion.

I Believe

The following are a few *presleep thoughts* to give your subconscious mind each night after you have finished your prayers.

By getting into the habit of repeating them to yourself night after night, you are instilling the essence of all religions into your subconscious mind. This technique of autosuggestion through autohypnosis gives you inner religion—a soul religion—a lifelong philosophy of life—a rock of Gibraltar *faith* in yourself.

1. *I believe* that life with all its complications is worth living.

2. *I believe* in the existence of a Higher Power, a Force of Love, that is eternal, that puts meaning into our lives.

3. *I believe* that I have the mind-power to survive all life's frustrations, disappointments, and misfortunes.

4. *I believe* that I have the capacity to acquire and experience inner peace of mind.

5. *I believe* that happiness comes from the ability to enjoy life and an unselfish desire to comfort and help others.

6. *I believe* that I am capable of improving my life by improving my way of thinking.

7. *I believe* that I can give love, accept love, and share love.

8. *I believe* that I can conquer any habit that is detrimental to my health.

9. *I believe* that I can apply all I have learned about myself and my subconscious mind toward making my life more successful.

10. *I believe* that life is what I make it, that I am master of my fate.

Remember that these are new attitudes that you are going to achieve and adopt. Jot them down on a small card and carry it with you all the time in your pocket or purse as you would your driver's license, identification or social security card. Label them "Daily Reminders." Refer to them daily. Soon you will be carrying out these printed self-given suggestions until you have them memorized. They can change your entire life from an old to a new and better way of thinking and living.

What to Remember

Self-hypnosis can help you develop the art of living a long, happy life. How? By giving yourself these posthypnotic suggestions. Believe them. Memorize them. Put them into practice:

1. I work to achieve and maintain my zest for life.
2. I make my own age.
3. Age is a state of mind.
4. I observe moderation in everything I do.
5. I take good care of my physical health.
6. I remain young in mind and heart by finding new pleasures, new interests, new friends.
7. I always seek to enjoy life and laugh more.
8. My goal in life is a longer, richer life.
9. I make all of my years interesting and meaningful.
10. I practice relaxation as a way of life.
11. Aging graciously means practicing being kind, unselfish, and understanding.
12. I release all worry, doubts, fears, and tensions.
13. I seek to grow wiser as I grow older.
14. A love of life, a gladness to be alive, a will to live will keep me young forever.
15. I always have a choice.

Richer Living Through New Thought Patterns

It is obviously our hope and recommendation that you put into practice what you have learned in this book. You will soon prove to yourself that life with all its varied complications can be rewarding—that life is worth living—that you can learn to master your fate through self-hypnosis.

In order to reassure ourselves that you will achieve whatever you had hoped to achieve from reading this book, let us summarize in this final chapter the important things we recommend that you keep in mind.

First, you now have an advantage over the average person because you have been educated in the *facts* about hypnosis. You have dispelled from your mind *fallacies* that would hamper you from benefiting from self-hypnosis. You know that self-hypnosis is a force for good, that there is nothing to fear from making good use of it. You can always rouse yourself from the hypnotic state. We also suggested in our early chapters that you exercise good judgment in consulting your physician or psychiatrist if there is any doubt in your mind as to whether your symptoms require medical attention or whether some deep-rooted emotional problem requires special management by a psychiatrist. We have found that giving our readers such advice is *essential*. We do not wish to convey the impression that self-hypnosis is a cure-all for anything and everything. By citing examples of conditions that responded favorably to self-hypnosis, we have shown specifically when self-hypnosis can be used effectively.

You should be convinced by now that self-hypnosis has unlimited potentialities. One of the most valuable benefits lies in the discovery of your inner self. Self-hypnosis can enable you to develop self-respect and self-confidence. It serves as a powerful weapon against self-defeatism. You can now view problems as temporary setbacks.

Now that you have learned the 4-A's method of self-hypnosis, apply it to specific problems. You will find that there will be almost nothing you cannot solve or correct. You'll experience personality maturity. You will learn to become immune to frustration. Your sense of values will be higher. You will automatically find yourself becoming the kind of a person you want to be. You will make better use of your time. Your thinking will be more systematized.

Self-hypnosis helps you develop self-discipline. It is a *self-teaching technique* for achieving your goals in life. By improving your *inner you*, through the better understanding of the subconscious, you experience a more successful relationship with other people.

Anyone can attain self-hypnosis because we are all *suggestible*— capable of being influenced by our own thinking. You remember we described hypnosis as a state of heightened suggestibility. When you induce the hypnotic state you are merely making yourself more *receptive* to suggestion—more receptive to *positive thinking* by utilizing the power of the subconscious mind and bypassing the critical factor of the conscious mind. Self-hypnosis makes use of conscious autosuggestion. But it goes a step beyond conscious thinking. It puts the subconscious mind to work, enabling it to accept and act on suggestions given to it by the conscious mind. Through self-hypnosis you can harness the potential and the force of your subconscious for constructive living. *This is the one great advantage over all other therapeutic methods of self-improvement.*

Self-hypnosis makes self-improvement a *lifelong habit*. You improve despite yourself. New thought patterns become a conditioned reflex. You change for the better *automatically*. Once you plant a seed in the ground it grows by itself. You can help it to grow faster by fertilizing the soil. Once you plant a thought in the subconscious mind it develops by itself into what might be called a *conditioned habit*.

One way of reminding your subconscious mind of the tremendous benefits derived from the use of self-hypnosis is to read and reread the many lists of self-suggestions in this book. In one of your sessions, after you are in the hypnotic state, review and memorize the essential substance of each chapter. In this way we guarantee that you will be getting the maximum value from the book.

You and Heredity

One of the most unfortunate and damaging fallacies that people still harbor is that nervousness, alcoholism, stubbornness, temper tantrums, and similar traits are inherited. Even those who have been enlightened by scientific knowledge and perhaps admit that these conditions are not really inherited, according to books they've read, handicap themselves by worrying about "heredity influences," what psychiatrists sometimes refer to as "hereditary predispositions."

Remember, we *imitate* consciously or unconsciously the traits of our parents, their way of thinking and doing things. In identifying ourselves with one or both parents, we grow up to be like them, not because of heredity but because of being exposed to their influences over the years. When we become adults we have an opportunity to reevaluate our parents in terms of personality assets and personality liabilities.

We no longer need to feel discouraged, thinking that we are chips off the old block, that "There's nothing I can do about the way I am," that "I must have taken after my father or my mother." We can change and modify those influences we attribute to our parents. Blaming our parents serves merely as a rationalization for not wanting to change ourselves for the better. It's nothing more than an alibi.

In attempting to achieve greater self-understanding through self-hypnosis, we can allow ourselves to regress to childhood and relive our early emotional relationship to our parents. Insight as to the origin of our present shortcomings can be helpful. But in psy-

choanalyzing our parents in our amateur way, we must suggest to
ourselves during self-hypnosis that we are going to be forgiving, that
we are not going to nurse resentments against our parents, that we
can undo any harm they might have done, that we can become our
new self by being *unlike* our parents, if need be. We can acquire an
entirely new personality via the method of self-suggestion.

It is comforting to have an eminent physician-writer such as Dr.
Walter Alvarez confess that he, too, was once a victim of a false
belief about heredity. He shared in his book, *Live at Peace with Your
Nerves*:

> When I was a young man I feared that I would not amount to
> much because I had inherited my mother's nervousness and fati-
> gability. I resolved that I would try to do the many wise and use-
> ful things my mother did, but avoid doing all the unwise things
> that wasted her strength and time.
>
> Obviously, my transformation did not come about overnight,
> but only after years of self-discipline. By hoarding my energies,
> I found enough strength for two jobs—one earning a living and
> the other doing research, writing, teaching and lecturing. I even
> had energy left over for a few hobbies, like mountain climbing,
> photography and book collecting.
>
> Once again we like to emphasize that the power of self-mastery
> lies with you. You have the mind-power to become what you
> want to be in spite of heredity, your family background, early
> environmental influences, or whatever. You can suggest away
> the notion that you are what your parents made you. Give your-
> self the suggestion instead that: "I am captain of my soul; I can
> achieve self-mastery through positive thinking, through self-
> hypnotic suggestions."

Making the Most of Each Day

There is much that can be said for the philosophy "Live one day at
a time." Wallowing in past regrets, or worrying about the future is
wasted energy. Concentrate on the *present*. (We don't wish to con-

tradict ourselves. Making plans for tomorrow, the next day, and the next is wise, but you must not forget that unless you start *today* with your self-improvement resolutions, the future will not be what you had hoped it to be. Tomorrow is dependent upon what you do today.) Discipline yourself to enjoy each moment of living. We don't know what tomorrow will bring. Self-hypnosis techniques can help you develop that feeling of being glad to be alive, that feeling that each new day is an interesting day, a day of growing, believing, a day of hope.

After reading a small paperback book entitled *Living Each Moment* by Ken Treiber, we had the pleasure of being introduced to the author and, much to our amazement, we learned that he is an engineer by profession. In our conversation with him, he told us that he practiced what he wrote. He was happy and enjoyed life and was inspired to tell others how he discovered this newfound happiness. We would like to pass on to our readers a few of the things he advocated and recommend that our readers incorporate them into their self-hypnosis sessions.

Here is his formula for happiness:

1. Obtain and maintain the best health possible.

2. Be honest.

3. Pay strict attention to the moment.

4. Have wholehearted interest in others.

5. Look for the good in everyone.

6. See each person as a precious being.

7. Be agreeable, not contrary.

8. Think about others rather than self.

9. Use the word "we" rather than "I."

10. Keep an open mind.

11. Don't be insulted if people disagree with you.

12. Let nothing disturb you.

13. Use your time wisely.

According to Treiber's diagram for achieving happiness, he claims if a person follows these rules he or she will possess:

1. Inward peace.
2. Ability to adjust to environment.
3. Joy of accomplishment.
4. Success.

These, in turn, will result in happiness.

There must be many others like Treiber who have discovered for themselves that they can have the kind of life they desire, a life inspired by achievements, a life of pleasantness and happiness.

Living can be simplified. You merely need to accept certain basic truths, certain fundamental commonsense rules, and utilize self-hypnosis as a means of putting these rules of healthier living into daily practice. If you begin today—now—the future will take care of itself. You can formulate your own rules for better living. Let them become part of a morning prayer that you recite to yourself at the beginning of each day.

Your own experience will be your best proof that self-hypnosis can accomplish wonders for you.

Twenty-five Guaranteed Dividends

Twenty-five guaranteed dividends from the use of self-hypnosis you can expect and are entitled to—if you follow carefully all of the instructions in the book:

1. It can change your way of living.
2. It can help you develop good health habits.
3. It can help you break bad habits.
4. It can help you reduce and achieve normal weight control.
5. It can help you stop smoking.
6. It can help you overcome addictive behavior.

7. It can help you overcome insomnia.

8. It can teach you to do everything the relaxed way.

9. It can help you overcome nervous tension.

10. It can help you eliminate chronic tiredness.

11. It can help you defeat mental depression and unhappy moods.

12. It can enable you to achieve a better sex life.

13. It can help you solve specific sexual problems, such as frigidity and impotence.

14. It can help you find love, accept love, give love, and share love.

15. It can help you develop a sense of humor, so essential to happier living.

16. It can help you enjoy life.

17. It can help you make more money and attain greater success in life.

18. It can help you control your emotions and relax away negative emotions such as anger, hate, selfishness, jealousy, vanity, and fear.

19. It can help you overcome feelings of inferiority and attain greater self-confidence.

20. It can give you a new lease on life.

21. It can help you get along better with others.

22. It can help you get along with yourself by acquiring a new personality.

23. It can help you stay young and live longer.

24. It can help you develop peace of mind.

25. It can help you develop a philosophy of life—that life at its worst is a fascinating experience—that it is wonderful to be alive—that people are basically good—that the world is improving—that we have the right to survive and enjoy life—that we have the right to be happy—that we *want, can, must,* and *will* achieve *better health, greater happiness, and more success.*

A Reinforced Suggestion

We suggested in our introduction that you can achieve many wonderful things with self-hypnosis. Now that you have completed reading the book, we hope you have been convinced that self-hypnosis can change your way of life, that you can become a healthier, happier person. However, we would like to be *reassured* that you have benefited from the contents of the book and recommend that you *reinforce* the following suggestions during one of your self-hypnotic therapy sessions:

> I was told at the beginning of the book that everyone has the capacity for self-improvement. Now that I have learned the technique of self-hypnosis, I will use it for the rest of my life as a valuable means of maintaining successful self-discipline.
>
> I am using it to help me achieve increasing emotional maturity and lasting peace of mind.
>
> I now have the formula for happiness and success.
>
> I read and reread this book as many times as is necessary so that I can continue to wisely apply the knowledge I have gained.
>
> I have discovered for myself that I have the power within me to control and influence my mind at will, that I can quickly convert negative thinking into positive thinking.
>
> Each day I remind myself that I am
>
> > Master of my Fate
> >
> > Captain of my Soul.

Chapter 18

Questions and Answers About Self-Hypnosis

In the many decades of our combined private practices, we have been asked many, many questions about self-hypnosis. Some of them may be questions that you, too, may have.

Where should I practice self-hypnosis?

Most people will want to find a quiet, private place for their initial sessions. When you are comfortable with the trance state, it is very likely that you will be able to do your self-hypnosis anywhere you choose, from waiting in line at the supermarket to sitting in a crowded airport. The most important environmental aspects for the beginner are comfort, security, and freedom from interruptions. If you absolutely cannot find such a place in your home, try sitting in your parked car. If you are in your office, close the door. Do the best you can, and you will find that there is always someplace where you can fulfill your new commitment to yourself.

How long should my session last?

The first few times, we recommend a relatively short session of about five minutes, just so you can acquaint yourself with the relaxed trance state. We strongly feel that you must be comfortable with the relaxation phase of the session before you attempt to do any serious change work on yourself. Keep in mind that even the shortest time of complete relaxation brings immediately gratifying results! You will probably work up to a session of 15 or 20 minutes within a couple of weeks. The more work you want to accomplish and the more complex your personal goals, the longer you may want to spend in your session. However, the more skilled you become at attaining relaxation, the less time you will spend in that phase. The amount of time that is best for you is something that only you can determine. Making it a habit is the key. Practice, practice, practice!

Should I sit up or lie down for my self-hypnosis session?

Unless your goal is to go to sleep, it is probably best for you to sit up comfortably in a chair that supports your back and perhaps even your head. Comfort is a personal, self-defined element you must determine for yourself.

I have always been told that "people never change," and when I look around me, I see a lot of evidence to support that. Can you comment?

You bet we can! You mentioned the evidence around you. Look again. Our world is in a constant state of change. Change is a natural part of our lives, as is obvious with the seasons, the tides, and the cycles of life and death of plants and animals. You may recall from Chapter 3 the fact that our bodies are continually renewing themselves on a cellular level. Expect to change. Make that expectation part of your daily philosophy of life. Tell yourself in your self-hypnosis sessions that you are seeing results now, and you will continue to improve each day.

How will I know that I've gone into hypnosis?

In spite of all the explanations and descriptions that we provide in the book, it seems that some people remain very reluctant to believe that they have indeed achieved the trance state. If you are one of those people, just be patient with yourself. The first few times you do it, you may not even be aware of it because the change from full waking consciousness to hypnotic consciousness can be very, very subtle. Notice how you become completely absorbed in the relaxation process. Notice also how your body responds to your suggestions of heaviness, lightness, warmth, and coolness. Observe where these feelings manifest in your body. Make a comparison of the way you felt when you started the session to the way you felt after you were done. Did more time pass than you thought? Time distortion is a good indicator of the hypnotic state. Once again, practice, practice, and practice!

What happens if an unexpected outside noise like a knock at the door or an airplane flying overhead happens when I am in the middle of my session?

You essentially have three choices in such circumstances. You can ignore the distraction, and just keep on doing what you're doing. Even if you are momentarily awakened, you can return to your hypnotic state in a very short time. You can also choose to use the noise as a part of your session. For instance, if the air-conditioner noise is noticeable to you, tell yourself, "The sounds of the air conditioner in the background are reminding me to relax more and more as I notice that just as the air temperature around me is changing, I am also making internal changes for the better." Sometimes you may just have to deal directly with the distraction. If you have an itch, scratch it. If you wonder who may be at your door, go open it. When you've handled the distraction, just return to your self-hypnosis. This is your session, and you are always in control.

How about prerecorded self-hypnosis tapes?

Some people do very well with prerecorded tapes. However, we believe that you will have the most success with a more personalized program using suggestions that are specific to you. If you want to use a prerecorded tape, why not just make one for yourself? You don't need any specialized, sophisticated equipment; a simple audio tape recorder will do. Your unconscious mind will certainly recognize and respond to your own voice than to someone else's. You can use a standard tape recorder. If you want to use relaxing music or environmental background sounds such as ocean waves or a gentle rain, do it. We encourage you to take any of the scripts or suggestions in this book and modify them in whatever way is suitable for you. You can easily edit your tapes as your program progresses, and as you become more and more skilled, you will very likely view the tapes as an option you may or may not want to continue to use.

What's the difference between hypnosis and the placebo effect?

Since hypnosis is so difficult to "pin down," or quantify, this is a difficult question to answer. We know that even though medical associations in both the U.S. and Great Britain acknowledge hypnosis as a valid therapeutic modality, scientists often look with skepticism at treatments that can't be explained. Some people believe that placebos function in a way that is very similar to hypnosis. This means that the unconscious mind is somehow stimulated by the placebo to respond in a specific way. While this may be true to some extent, there are also some notable differences. Surely you've heard of people getting "cured" when they thought they were being given a new drug, only to relapse when they find out it was a sugar pill. Belief is the critical element in such a case. However, you do not have to believe in hypnosis for it to be effective. For hypnosis to work, all that is needed is the genuine desire to achieve a goal and the commitment to be persistent in its achievement. With a placebo, the unconscious is somehow "fooled" into believing the source of the help, such as a pill or a lotion, is coming from outside the self. With hypnosis, the responsibility and control is with you. There is no trickery or deception. It is your own motivation, desire, and dedication that cause the change to take place. In the end, we do not have to understand why something happens to enjoy the benefits of it. Such is the case with electricity and countless other phenomena. Such is also the case with hypnosis. It is a remarkable tool that works, and that's all you really need to know to begin to enjoy its help.

I am able to accomplish the relaxed state you describe in Step 1, Autorelaxation. However, I feel like sometimes I would enjoy an even deeper feeling of relaxation. Is this possible?

First of all, we want you to be clear that a light trance state is all that is necessary for your subconscious mind to assimilate the autotherapy suggestions you provide in Step 4. However, if you wish to accomplish an even deeper trance state, you can use what hypnotherapists refer to as "deepening techniques." We will give you a few here that we have adapted from our own practice. Consider them completely optional. Use one or more of them during the autorelaxation phase of your self-hypnosis session, after you have done your basic autorelaxation.

> **Visual Imagery Technique**—This is one of the best and easiest-to-use techniques for deepening the trance state. Just imagine any scene that means "peaceful" to you. For example, see yourself comfortable in your bed, lying down and sleeping deeply. Perhaps you would rather be stretched out under a summer sun at the beach or swinging back and forth in a hammock. Just imagine the scene, and feel yourself going deeper and deeper with each breath.

> **Escalator Technique**—Imagine yourself riding down an elevator or an escalator. Start counting backward slowly to yourself from 20 to zero. Tell yourself that the further down you go on the elevator or escalator, the deeper you will go into a hypnotic state.

> **Counting Method**—Count forward to 100 or backward from 100. You may choose to count by ones, twos, fives, whatever you wish. Tell yourself that with each number, you will be more relaxed.

> **Hand Levitation**—Suggest to yourself that it is time for your hand to rise from your lap, and imagine that as it rises, your arm lifts your hand until it gently touches your face. As soon as you feel your fingers touch your face, your arm will immediately become heavy and fall to your thigh. As this happens, you go deeper into hypnosis than ever before.

What happens if I get sleepy or drowsy while trying to bring on the hypnotic state?

If your body is tired, and you relax it completely, you may well fall into a natural sleep. You would wake up just as you always do from a nap. However, if it is your goal to achieve more energy and alertness, then tell yourself before you begin the relaxation process that you intend to increase your energy and that you will awaken from your session with renewed vigor and feeling more alert.

Can self-hypnosis be used to improve children's schoolwork or test taking?

Yes. Children make some of the best self-hypnotic subjects because of their ability to imagine. Most of them also have a great capacity to picture things in their minds. There are many self-hypnosis suggestions in this book that can be adapted to individual children. The main thing to teach them is to "see yourself as . . . [successful, concentrating, remembering, calm, relaxed, tension-free, etc.]." Self-hypnosis is an excellent study tool for children. Teach your children how to use this skill. It is a gift that they will use for a lifetime.

Can someone who is easily distracted learn to use self-hypnosis?

If a person wants to learn self-hypnosis, it is entirely possible. There are people who have a difficult time concentrating on one thing because they have "busy" minds that are accustomed to flitting from one topic to another. The best way to deal with this situation is to use a counting technique that is modified specifically for use with such "resistant" subjects. It follows here:

> I am beginning to count to myself, and I will count from zero to the number 20. I will begin with my eyes open, close them on the next count, open them on the following, close them again on the next, and repeat this procedure again and again. (Zero . . . eyes open . . . one . . . eyes closed . . . two . . . eyes open . . . three . . . eyes closed . . . four . . . eyes open, and so forth.) With each count, my eyes will become heavier and heavier and my body will relax more and more. Presently my eyes will remain closed, and I fall until my eyes will not open any longer.

Is it safe to use self-hypnosis in public places?

It is always "safe" to use self-hypnosis because you are always in control. Your conscious mind and the critical factor we discussed earlier will always intervene in the event of danger or emergency. However, it seems unlikely that you would choose to relax and enter a self-hypnotic trance while you are walking down the street or in the middle of a room full of people. You will very likely, however, use the post-hypnotic suggestions you have given yourself in your prior, planned self-hypnosis sessions to change or alter your behavior or perceptions in public places. In that sense, you are indeed using self-hypnosis in a public place. Another example of an appropriate public use of self-hypnosis would be when you need to summon a sense of calm, a feeling of confidence, or a surge of energy. When you've mastered the basics, you will have the ability to do any of those things and more in a very short time whenever and wherever you want.

I still have an issue with control. Even though I understand that this is self-hypnosis, I somehow feel like I'm giving something up. Does that sound crazy?

Control is a big issue with a lot of people, and we consider it to be a perfectly sane question! You may have a misunderstanding that was borne out of seeing someone in a stage hypnosis show behaving in some ridiculous way. You may fear losing the memory of what happens during the self-hypnosis session. Perhaps you still harbor some idea that you will have a difficult time returning to full waking consciousness. All of these ideas are related to control, and they are common misconceptions about hypnosis. Please review Chapter 1 about the facts and fallacies of hypnosis. If you approach your self-hypnosis with an open mind and a belief that it will help you, you will demonstrate to yourself that you are not giving anything up. On the contrary, you are gaining a lot.

To be truthful, sometimes I want to change, and sometimes I just don't. Can self-hypnosis help?

Being truthful with yourself is very important. Self-hypnosis can help you only if you really want it to help you. If you have little or no desire to change, you are sure to be a poor subject for self-hypnosis therapy. Many people are not ready to give up their habits or undesirable behavior. Motivation is the single most important element in a successful self-hypnosis experience. Instead of approaching self-hypnosis with the idea of change, why not just begin to use it for relaxation? Everyone can benefit from that. When you're confident that change is what you desire, you will have mastered the first essential step, autorelaxation.

How does the medical community feel about hypnosis?

That's an excellent question to which we can only offer a rather ambiguous answer: It depends on whom you ask. Even though the American Medical Association recognized hypnosis as a "viable therapeutic modality" in the mid-1950s, a lot of physicians—including psychiatrists—scoff at hypnosis. This is probably due to prejudice incurred during their medical training or even too much exposure to Hollywood's version of hypnosis. Another contributing factor is that until recently, the mind-body connection was not recognized as a "scientific" fact, and doctors or therapists that dabbled in such things did so at the peril of their professional peer status. However, there have always been doctors who were willing to go against the thinking of the mainstream medical community to explore new methods of healing. Such people who may have been considered "weird" in the past are frequently considered innovators today.

I would really like to visit a professional hypnotherapist. Can you give me some direction about how I can find a good one?

First, visit a medical doctor and have a thorough checkup. It is important that you make sure that your problem is not one that really needs medical attention. If you are severely depressed or have other serious mental complaints, see a medical doctor that specializes in psychiatry or a licensed psychotherapist. If your physician determines that you do indeed need medical attention, you can still see a hypnotherapist if you have a written referral from a medical doctor or a licensed psychotherapist. Once you have determined you have no medical problems, or if you have your referral, you should have no trouble finding a competent hypnotherapist in your area. You have several options: Ask your doctor or psychologist for a recommendation, or look in the yellow pages of your telephone directory under "Hypnosis" and call your local chapter of the American Society of Clinical Hypnosis. Another excellent option is to contact the American Board of Hypnotherapy (ABH), one of the largest professional hypnotherapy organizations in the world. The ABH maintains a database of thousands of its members and can give you the name and telephone number of a certified hypnotherapist in your area, as well as the hypnotherapist's training, background, experience, and specialty. You can reach the ABH at one of their toll-free telephone numbers: 800-634-9766 or 800-872-9996.

Epilogue

We predict techniques in hypnosis and self-hypnosis will occupy an important place in our daily lives in the not-too-distant future.

J. B. S. Haldane, the famous British biologist, obviously shared this same point of view, as evidenced by his statement:

> Anyone who has seen even a single example of the power of hypnosis and suggestion must realize that the face of the world and the possibilities of existence will be totally altered when we can control their effects and standardize their application.

We believe that hypnosis has potentials that are unlimited and is destined to become a great force in our society. Most people will, in the future, be practicing the techniques of self-hypnosis, for the breaking of bad habits, the control of one's emotions, the improvement of one's health and personality, and the accomplishment of our various goals in life.

Self-hypnosis will become the *master key to successful living*.

The Best Autorelaxation/ Induction Procedures for You to Hypnotize Yourself

Before deciding upon—and practicing—one of the following induction procedures, you may wish to review the section in Chapter 5 about autorelaxation. Since the relaxation component is the first, most important part of the process, you may find that one "script" is more to your liking than another is. We have compiled here a few alternative relaxation scripts that are yours to use anytime you wish. Perhaps you would like to record your favorite on an audiocassette to play back whenever you need a relaxation break or even as a part of your regular self-hypnosis session.

Autorelaxation/Induction Optional Procedure #1

I am letting all the muscles of my body become loose and limp. My breathing is settling into an easy, natural, even and rhythmical pattern. And as I do this I can feel myself gradually beginning to relax more and more. With each breath that I breathe I am becoming more and more relaxed and every muscle in my body is becoming more and more comfortable. And as I breathe more slowly, more evenly, I am settling down more and more into a wonderful, comfortable feeling. There is nothing for me to do, no one to bother me, no work to be done and I am free just to settle back, breathe easily and rhythmically, and I will gradually feel more and more relaxation spreading downward from the top of my head to the tops of my toes. Every muscle, every fiber, every bone of my body is gradually being drained of all tension and all stress and I am sinking—deeper—and—deeper—into a wonderful state of pleasant and comfortable relaxation.

The muscles of my eyes are feeling more relaxed now and it seems as though my eyelids almost flutter. The flesh on my face is beginning to droop—and gradually, as I continue to breathe easily and rhythmically, the flesh on my cheeks seems to hang heavy from my cheekbones. And my jaw seems slack now—even my tongue is relaxed.

Very gradually I feel my neck muscles going limp, and my head feels heavy now, and I let it lean wherever it is comfortable.

The relaxation is spreading outward from my neck now, moving slowly across my shoulders so that my shoulders are losing their muscle tone and are feeling very, very loose. I can feel the stress draining down my upper arms now, followed by a pleasant sense of comfortable relaxation flowing down my upper arms and through my elbows and down through my forearms to my wrists and hands. I feel a tingling in my hands and fingers now as all the stress drains down and off the ends of my fingers and is gone.

Every muscle, every fiber, every nerve of my face, my neck, my shoulders, and my arms—now relaxed and very, very comfortable.

It is curious that my chest muscles are relaxing now, too, and the muscles of my stomach and abdomen are becoming limp and relaxed—as every nerve, every fiber, every muscle of my body lets go.

The muscles of my back from my shoulders to my hips are also limp.

My hips and thighs are relaxing, too, as all the stress of my entire body drains down and is replaced by a warm flow of comfortable relaxation that moves gradually down through my thighs, passing through and filling the calves of my legs and goes down through my ankles to my feet, which also have that tingling sensation as all the stress of my entire body drains down and off the ends of my toes—and is gone.

All the muscles of my entire body are now in a very comfortable state of relaxed equilibrium.

As I am noticing and feeling myself becoming more comfortable and more relaxed, it is wonderful to observe how pleasant—how agreeable—this state of relaxation is.

And as I continue to enjoy this relaxation, I imagine a staircase, and I see myself stand at the top of this staircase, looking down. I know there are 20 steps but I see only whatever is comfortable for me to see. But I do notice that the steps are covered with a deep silencing [insert your favorite color here] carpet that assures restful quietness. The stair rail is a beautiful, polished wood that feels so cool and smooth to my touch.

I am going to go down this staircase—one—step—at—a—time. And as I go down each step, I will notice how I feel just a bit more comfortable.

One step down the staircase.

Two steps down the staircase.

Three steps down the staircase.

I am feeling more comfortable now. I realize that I can pay attention to anything I like, but it's easier to listen to these relaxing words as they pass through my mind and notice how easy it is to understand their meaning as I continue to feel more and more comfortable.

Four steps down the staircase—with nothing to do, no one to bother me as I gradually sink—deeper—and—deeper—and become more and more comfortable.

Five steps down the staircase. One quarter of the way down now—beginning to feel even more comfortable as I notice how pleasant that feeling is that flows over me as I move down.

Six steps down the staircase. I notice that sounds that once were distracting are less distracting now—in fact, it seems as though every distraction fades further and further into the distance—and there is nothing to bother me—nothing to disturb me.

Seven steps down the staircase—all distractions fade further and further into the distance and they don't matter any more.

Eight steps down the staircase. There is nothing to bother me, nothing to disturb me, and I am going deeper and deeper into a feeling of more comfort and more relaxation.

Deeper—and—deeper—and it is wonderful to observe that I am moving slowly into a very deep state of relaxed twilight awareness.

Halfway down the staircase—feeling more and more relaxed and more and more comfortable.

Eleven steps down the staircase—and I feel myself drifting even deeper—way down now—deeper and deeper into a very deep state of relaxed comfort.

Twelve steps down the staircase. I notice a sense of becoming more and more listless, even a feeling of absolute drowsiness and my body feels deeply relaxed.

So very comfortable.

Fourteen steps down the staircase. My breathing is still rhythmically and restfully even and I am so naturally relaxed.

Three-quarters of the way down the staircase completely relaxed now.

Deeper and deeper relaxed.

Seventeen steps down the staircase—with nothing to bother me, nothing to disturb me as I continue to enjoy increasing comfort and deep relaxation.

Eighteen steps down the staircase—almost to the bottom. Wondering what I will experience at the bottom of the staircase. Thinking perhaps nothing more than increasing comfort, composure, and relaxation. Knowing there is nothing to bother me—nothing to disturb me.

And now—I let it all sink down, composed, comfortable, and relaxed. And I am so pleased to notice, as I let myself keep on sinking deeper and deeper, that increased composure, comfort, and relaxation are spreading and deepening with each breath I take, so that my body is becoming more and more comfortable. I just remain calm noticing the comfort and attending effortlessly to these relaxing thoughts.

The final step on the staircase, I am here on the landing at the bottom of the staircase and I am so pleasantly and completely relaxed.

And now I can enjoy this state of deep relaxation and recall that I have experienced this wonderful relaxation before. It is such a natural and refreshingly restful feeling. And I can experience this relaxed feeling again anytime I wish. All I have to do is to repeat this induction procedure, follow the instructions and suggestions, and I will find it easier and easier each time. And as I repeat this induction procedure over and over, preferably twice each day, this composed comfortable relaxation will become an experience I can call up any time I so desire.

(At this point you may either (a) quietly enjoy your relaxed state for a time, or (b) quietly repeat the positive suggestions you earlier prepared, knowing that they will be directly implanted in your subconscious mind. They then become permanently imprinted in your memory bank to be yielded up to your conscious mind as powerful aids in achieving that happiness and success you desire.)

And in a moment—but not yet—I am going to count from twenty to one, and when I begin to count I will slowly and comfortably come back up the staircase feeling myself becoming more and more alert with each step so that when I reach step number three, my eyes will be ready to open. And when I reach step number two, my eyes will be open, and when I reach step number one, my eyes will be open wide and I will be alert, confident, and notice how much more relaxed I feel—as though I have had a quiet comfortable nap—knowing that I am free—free to repeat this wonderful deep self-hypnotic relaxation experience anytime I wish.

And now—counting my way back up the staircase . . . 20—19—18—17—16—15—feeling wonderful—14—13—12—11—10—halfway up the staircase feeling more and more alert and confident—9—8—7—6—5—4—3—my eyes are almost ready to open—2—my eyes are open—1 . . . my eyes are open wide and I feel wonderfully wide awake.

Autorelaxation/Induction Optional Procedure #2

In this procedure you will begin the relaxation process with your feet and work upward. Start by taking a deep breath and exhaling it slowly, and as you allow your breathing to settle into an easy, natural, even and rhythmical pattern, you should concentrate on your feet, thinking the following thoughts to yourself:

I feel a slight tingling sensation in my feet as they begin to relax and I can feel them gradually becoming more and more relaxed. There seems to be a warm heaviness that is beginning to flow through them as they become more relaxed. And this flow of warm, soothing relaxation is starting to gradually move from my feet up through my ankles and into the calves of my legs, and as it does I can feel my muscles gradually feeling heavier and heavier—so comfortably relaxed. The flow of that warm relaxed sensation is moving through my knees now—and into and filling the muscles of my thighs. My legs are feeling heavier and heavier now and feel so very comfortably relaxed.

It is interesting to me that my hands are now feeling that tingling sensation, too. I notice that same comfortable feeling flowing into my hands and spreading its soothing warmth up through my wrists to encompass my forearms. And it feels so enjoyable as it spreads into my upper arms and leaves my arms, like my legs, feeling so limp and so very, very comfortable.

My shoulders are going loose now, too, and the relaxation is spreading to the muscles of my stomach and abdomen. A pleasant warmth and relaxation that is moving up through my neck muscles so that they, too, are becoming relaxed and limp are inundating my entire body. And my jaws are going slack—I can feel my jaws becoming loose and heavy. My tongue feels relaxed, and the flesh on my face is beginning to droop and gradually seems to hang heavy from my cheekbones. My eyes are so comfortably drowsy now and my eyelids so heavy. It feels so good to be relaxed. Even the skin on my forehead is smoothing out and I feel so quiet, so comfortably relaxed, and so inwardly calm.

Every muscle of my entire body is in a wonderful state of relaxed equilibrium and I feel so peacefully comfortable and relaxed.

With every breath that I breathe I can feel myself going deeper and deeper into an even greater depth of relaxation—and there is nothing to bother me, nothing to disturb me. Sounds that were once distracting are no longer distracting and they seem to fade further and further into the distance and they don't matter anymore.

In a moment, when I count to five, I will feel myself going into a much deeper relaxation—deeper than I have ever been before, always aware of these relaxing thoughts with all else fading further and further into the distance.

ONE—Beginning to drift deeper.

TWO—Away down now—so comfortable.

THREE—Deeper and deeper relaxed.

FOUR—So calm, so quiet, so comfortable.

FIVE—Away down now, deeper and deeper relaxed.

And now, while this relaxation continues to deepen throughout my body and I breathe so easily and rhythmically, it is wonderful to realize that I can enjoy this pleasant, relaxed, warm, and comfortable sensation anytime I choose. All I have to do is to repeat this procedure and I will achieve this quiet peaceful state of twilight awareness. And since I know that when I am relaxed like this my subconscious mind is most accessible to me, I can now plant positive suggestions in it and they will become permanently imprinted in my memory bank to give me powerful assistance in becoming that happy and successful person I have always wanted to be.

(At this point you can repeat quietly to yourself those positive suggestions that you have worked out earlier.)

And in a moment—but not yet—I am going to count from ten to zero, and as I do I will come back up to full alertness. I will continue to feel internally calm and have a wonderful feeling of satisfaction and confidence—and when I get to number two, my eyes will be almost ready to open, and when I get to number one, my eyes will open, and when I get to zero, my eyes will be open wide and I be fully alert and feel wonderfully refreshed as though I have had a short nap.

Counting now—10—9—8—7—gradually feeling more alert—6—5—feeling wonderful—4—3—2—my eyes are almost ready to open—1—my eyes are open—and 0—my eyes are open wide and I am alert, refreshed, and feeling wonderful.

Autorelaxation/Induction Optional Procedure #3

As I breathe easily and naturally, I can feel myself gradually beginning to relax. Each breath that I breathe enables me to relax more and more, and every muscle in my body is becoming more and more comfortable. And as I breathe more slowly, more evenly, I am settling down into a wonderful comfortable feeling. There is nothing for me to do, no one to disturb me, no work to be done and I am free just to settle back, breathe easily and rhythmically, and I am gradually feeling more comfortable, and I feel relaxation spreading downward progressively from the top of my head to the tips of my toes. Every muscle, every fiber, every nerve in my body is gradually being drained of all tension and all stress and I am sinking—deeper—and—deeper—into a wonderful state of pleasant and comfortable relaxation.

And now I am picturing the face of a clock—a large clock with a white face. The numbers on the white clock face are black. There is only one hand on the clock, it is the big hand, it is black and it is pointing straight up to number twelve.

In a moment—but not yet—this hand will begin to move counterclockwise, going slowly from twelve all the way around to one and up to its upright position again. And as the hand passes each number, that number will disappear from the face of the clock—and as each number disappears, I will feel my present state of comfortable relaxation deepen and I will become more and more comfortable and more and more deeply relaxed. When all of the numbers on the face of the clock are gone and the face is blank, I will be completely relaxed and in a wonderful state of twilight awareness—ready at that point to silently give my subconscious mind those positive suggestions which will be powerful aids to me in achieving happiness and success.

And now, I am picturing very vividly the white face of my clock with the big hand pointing to twelve. The big hand is beginning to move slowly toward number eleven and as it moves away from twelve that number disappears and the space is blank, and as the hand continues to move slowly and twelve vanishes, I seem to be drifting into more relaxation.

The hand is passing eleven now and eleven is gone, too—and my relaxation is deepening with each breath that I breathe. And as ten is approached and passed and disappears I am sinking into a quiet listlessness. The hand is approaching nine and as it moves slowly and silently by, nine goes away and I go deeper and deeper into a more comfortable relaxation. Number eight is coming up and there it goes, too, as the hand moves by, and as I breathe easily and naturally I am drifting into a very pleasant drowsiness. Silently the hand comes to seven, passes it, and seven is gone. Number six is being approached and as the hand moves slowly by, number six is gone, too. One half of the clock face is blank now and I am becoming more and more drowsy as the hand passes five and five has vanished. Very deeply relaxed now, so peaceful, so still, so calm. Number four just disappeared as the hand passed over it and moves on to number three—and three is gone. Slowly and quietly the hand comes up to two and wipes off number two. The clock face is almost blank now and I am deeply relaxed and in that pleasant state of twilight awareness as the hand reaches and passes number one, and with the disappearance of number one the clock face is completely blank—there is nothing to disturb me, and I am so comfortably calm and relaxed.

While my subconscious mind is so readily accessible I will take this restful time to place my positive suggestions in it, knowing they will be acceptable and be imprinted in my memory bank to be available to give me powerful assistance in achieving my goals.

(At this point present your previously prepared positive suggestions.)

And now I am clearly picturing the blank face of my clock again. The big hand is still facing straight up. In a moment the hand will begin to move clockwise and as it does the numbers will reappear in order and I will gradually become more alert. And as number ten appears I will almost open my eyes—at number eleven my eyes will open, and as the big hand returns to twelve I will be alert, confident, and perhaps notice how much more refreshed I feel as though I have had a quiet, refreshing nap.

Watching the blank face of my clock I see the big hand beginning to move to the right, and as it passes five minutes after the hour, number one reappears. Gradually moving and passing ten minutes after one, the number two reappears. The hand is still moving and number three reappears and then number four and, in time, number five and number six. I am feeling calm and confident as number seven reappears and the hand moves on past eight—feeling wonderful as number nine reappears. I am starting to feel more aware of my surroundings, more relaxed and alert, almost ready to open my eyes as number ten appears. There is number eleven and my eyes are open, and as twelve comes up I am alert, confident, and feeling wonderful.

Autorelaxation Optional Procedure #4

The following induction procedure begins with the familiar pattern employed in the previous procedure but is then shortened. Some people may find this more concise induction procedure more suitable for them. Should you try this procedure and find it not as effective at first, you can lengthen it by repeating the count. Begin by closing your eyes to shut out all visual distractions.

As I breathe easily and naturally, I am gradually beginning to relax more and more. With each breath that I breathe I am becoming increasingly relaxed, and every muscle of my body is becoming more and more comfortable. And as I breathe more slowly, more evenly, I am settling down more and more into a wonderfully deep and comfortable feeling. There is nothing for me to do, no one to disturb me and I am free just to settle back, breathe easily and rhythmically, and gradually feel more and more comfortable. And I can feel more and more relaxation spreading gradually downward from the top of my head to the tips of my toes. Every muscle, every nerve, every fiber of my entire body is gradually being drained of all tension and all stress, and I am sinking deeper and deeper into a wonderfully drowsy state of pleasant and comfortable relaxation that I enjoy more and more. When I count to five I will go into a deeper and more pleasant state of twilight awareness than I have ever experienced before. Counting now . . . one . . . breathing easily and rhythmically and drifting deeper . . . two . . . away down—deeper—deeper—twice as deep as ever before. Three . . . more and more relaxation is spreading throughout my entire body and I am going twice as deep as ever before. Four . . . drifting pleasantly deeper and deeper . . . and five . . . way down now, deeper than I have ever been before. Every muscle, every nerve, every fiber from the top of my head to the tips of my toes is so comfortably relaxed and I am sinking deeper and deeper into a wonderfully drowsy twilight state of pleasant and comfortable relaxation.

And now, while this comfort and relaxation deepens and spreads throughout my entire body, I will give my subconscious those positive suggestions which will be powerful aids to me in becoming that happy and successful person I want to be.

(At this point present the previously prepared positive suggestions. When you are ready to return to complete alertness, continue with the following.)

As I count from ten to zero I will gradually return to full alertness. When I reach number two, my eyes will feel like opening, and when I reach number one, my eyes will open. When I reach zero, my eyes will be open wide, and I will be alert and feel refreshed as though I have just had a restful nap.

Counting—10—9—8—7—6—beginning to be more alert—5—4—3—feeling wonderful—2—my eyes feel like opening now—1—my eyes are open—and 0—my eyes are open wide and I feel rested, alert, and wonderful.

Autorelaxation Optional Procedure #5

In this induction procedure you will begin with experiencing feelings of relaxation in your hands and proceeding from there. The initial preparation is always the same. Make yourself comfortable, close your eyes, breathe easily and naturally, relax all the muscles of your body, and focus your full attention on the flow of thoughts as follows:

My hands are beginning to feel more and more relaxed. Little by little, as I breathe easily and rhythmically, my hands are becoming more and more relaxed. They feel more limp now and are becoming heavier and heavier. They seem, in fact, to feel like warm, wet gloves, heavy and limp. And this feeling of warm relaxation is beginning to spread up through my wrists and into my forearms so that my hands and forearms are more and more comfortably heavy and relaxed. And as I let go, the muscles of my upper arms experience this same comfortable relaxation spreading through my elbows and flowing into the muscles of both my entire arms. And as I keep letting go and enjoying this relaxation my shoulders are drooping and becoming very loose and comfortably relaxed. Gradually, as I breathe easily and rhythmically, my entire body is being filled with a wonderful peacefulness and a quiet, restful, inner calm that deepens and grows with each breath that I breathe—so comfortable, so peacefully serene, so relaxed.

The muscles of my neck are letting go, too, now and becoming very limp and loose. My jaw is becoming slack. Even my tongue is relaxed. The skin on my face is beginning to relax and even seems to hang heavy from my cheek as every muscle, every nerve, and every fiber of my entire body lets go and is filled with a wonderful sense of comfort, relaxation, and peace. The skin between my eyes is relaxing and the little lines at the corners of my eyes are smoothing out. My eyes are drowsy and my eyelids so pleasantly heavy.

And as I continue to breathe easily and naturally, I am drifting deeper and deeper into an ever-deepening relaxation, and a wonderful inner calm and satisfying peace is flowing into me as I enjoy a pleasantly serene state of twilight awareness.

And now, while my subconscious mind is receptively accessible, I will feed it the positive suggestions which will be nourished and grow to be powerful influences in moving me forward toward success and the achievement of my goals.

(At this point present your previously prepared positive suggestions, and when you are ready to return to full alertness, continue.)

And now—as I count from ten to zero I will gradually return to full alertness. When I reach number two, my eyes will be almost ready to open, and when I reach number one, my eyes will be open, and when I reach zero, my eyes will be open wide and I will be alert and feel refreshed as though I have had a pleasant nap.

Counting—10—9—8—the heaviness is drifting away—7—6—beginning to feel more alert—5—4—feeling wonderful—3—2—my eyes are almost ready to open—1—my eyes are open—and 0—my eyes are open wide and I am alert, wide awake, and feeling wonderful.

Autorelaxation Optional Procedure #6

In this induction procedure you should begin by keeping your eyes open. The usual conditions of making yourself comfortable and free from distractions should be observed. With your eyes open, just stare at a fixed point. This can be a lighted candle or a thumbtack in the wall—or any point you choose in the room where you are. As you stare at this point allow the muscles of your eyes to be relaxed, even if this means that what you are staring at becomes blurred, or even results in double vision. The more relaxed your eye muscles, the better overall relaxation you will experience. As you remain relaxed and staring at the object you have chosen, begin to concentrate on your eyes and eyelids. Notice how they are gradually becoming tired and heavy. Think of this fatigue and heaviness in your eyelids, and after two or three minutes, maybe more, you will find it more and more difficult to hold your eyes open. When you reach this point, allow your eyes to close, and think to yourself the following flow of thoughts:

It feels so good to close my eyes. My eyelids are so heavy, so relaxed, and they feel so comfortable when closed. Their relaxation is gradually spreading to the rest of my face. My face feels relaxed as the muscles around my eyes and mouth become loose and limp.

The relaxation is spreading down through my neck muscles now so that my head begins to feel heavy and I let it lean where it is most comfortable. The relaxation is spreading slowly out from my neck across my shoulders and my shoulders are losing their muscle tone and feeling very loose and relaxed. Now the relaxation is flowing down my upper arms through my elbows to my forearms and on down through my wrists to my hands and fingers, which have that tingling sensation as all the tension and stress drain off the ends of my fingers and are gone.

Every muscle and every fiber of my head, my neck, my shoulders, and my arms is relaxed now and I feel so pleasantly comfortable and relaxed.

My chest muscles are relaxing, too, and this relaxation is spreading downward to the muscles of my stomach and abdomen.

And the muscles of my back, from my shoulders to my hips, are going limp—I can feel this. My hips and thighs are feeling a flow of relaxing warmth spreading downward, filling the muscles of my thighs and passing on down and flooding the muscles of the calves of my legs. And as this relaxation moves through my ankles, to my feet and toes, I can feel that tingling sensation as all the tension of my entire body drains down and off the ends of my toes and is gone.

Every muscle in my body is now in a wonderful state of relaxed equilibrium.

With every breath that I breathe I can feel myself going into a deeper and deeper state of wonderful relaxation. There is no one to bother me, nothing to disturb me. Sounds that were once distracting are no longer bothersome at all, and they seem to fade further and further into the distance. They just don't matter any more.

When I count to five, I will feel myself drift deeper with each digit I say, and all distractions will fade further and further away.

ONE—beginning to drift deeper and deeper.

TWO—way down—so relaxed and so comfortable.

THREE—deeper and deeper relaxed.

FOUR—so peacefully quiet, comfortable, and calm.

FIVE—way down now, deeper and even deeper relaxed.

(At this point you can quietly repeat to yourself those positive suggestions that you have written out earlier. When you are ready to return to full alertness, you can continue as follows.)

When I count from five to zero, I will gradually return to full alertness. I will continue to feel internally calm and will have a continuing feeling of confidence and optimism. When I get to number two, my eyes will be almost ready to open, and when I get to number one, my eyes will open, and when I reach zero, my eyes will be open wide and I will feel relaxed, confident, and rested as though I have just taken a relaxing nap.

Counting now—5—4—becoming more alert—3—feel wonderful—2—my eyes are almost ready to open—1—my eyes are open—
and 0—my eyes are open wide and I feel wonderful.

Dr. Masud Ansari's Subjective Technique

Sit in a comfortable chair or lie down on a couch or bed; fix your
eyes on a spot on the wall above eye level or on the ceiling. Focus
your attention on your eyelids. Imagine that your eyelids are becoming very heavy. Feel this heaviness. Again and again, mentally tell
yourself:

> *My eyes are getting very heavy. I feel my eyes getting very heavy
> and the heavier they become, the more comfortable and relaxed
> I feel. It seems that it is becoming impossible for me to keep my eye-
> lids open. It really feels so good to close my eyes. I will count to
> three. When I complete the count, it will be absolutely impossible
> for me to keep my eyelids open. It really feels so good to close my
> eyes. I will count to three. When I complete the count, it will be
> completely impossible for me to keep my eyes open. ONE . . . my
> eyes are narrowing to a slit. They are about to close. TWO . . . my
> eyelids are dropping. THREE . . . they are closing, they are closing
> . . . they are closing.*

Then tell yourself:

> *My eyelids are now locked together; they are stuck fast, so tight-
> ly stuck that I cannot open them. Now I just stop trying to open
> them. I can open my eyes whenever I choose, but I want to keep
> them closed for now.*

Now think of the following peaceful scene: Imagine you are
walking around a swimming pool in the middle of a beautiful garden. It is mid-spring. The weather is very pleasant. It is three o'clock
in the afternoon. You keep walking alongside the pool. All around
the pool are red, white, and yellow roses. A fragrant group of beautiful blooming bushes are close by. A mild breeze blows across the

pool, and it brings with it the lovely scent of the flowers. You keep walking by, carrying with you the memory of that nice fragrance. You look ahead of you and spot a hammock stretched between two shady trees. You decide to lie down in that hammock in the midst of the beautiful garden and enjoy your deep relaxation. So you approach the hammock and lie down in its folds, and you love its comfort. As the hammock sways back and forth, back and forth, you feel yourself becoming even more deeply relaxed. Back and forth, deeper and deeper.

When you are ready, give yourself the suggestions that you have prepared ahead of time. Then you make the suggestions to yourself that you are ready to return to normal waking consciousness.

Spiegel's Relaxation Technique

Psychiatrists Herbert and David Spiegel developed another interesting self-hypnosis method to teach to their patients:

> *Sit or lie down, and to yourself, count to three. At one, you do one thing; at two, you do two things; and at three, you do three things. In all, you carry out six things. At one, look up toward your eyebrows; at two, while looking up, close your eyelids and take a deep breath; and at three, exhale, let your eyes relax, and let your body float. As you feel yourself floating, you permit one hand or the other to feel like a buoyant balloon and let it float upward. When it reaches this upright position, it becomes the signal for you to enter a state of meditation. This floating sensation signals your mind to turn inward and pay attention to your own thoughts—like private meditation. Ballet dancers and athletes float all the time. That is why they concentrate and coordinate their movements so well. When they do not float, they are tense and do not do as well.*

The Spiegels tell their patients that in the beginning, they should do these exercises as often as ten times a day, preferably every one or two hours. At first, the exercises take a minute, but as patients become more adept, they can do it in much less time. Then the

Speigels tell their patients to awaken themselves with the following method of counting backward:

> *Now* three, *get ready;* two, *with your eyelids closed, roll up your eyes; and* one, *let your eyelids open slowly. Then when your eyes are back in focus, slowly make a fist with the hand that is up, and as you open your fist slowly, your usual sensation and control returns. Let your hand float downward.*

A p p e 2 *n d i x*

Exercises in Imagery and Awareness

Your ability to experience imagery and be aware of that experience is a major determinant in your success with self-hypnosis. Imagery is a skill that some people seem to have naturally while others have to work a little harder to "see" pictures in their minds. Being aware just means paying attention. We think that you will find the following exercises useful in helping you to develop the skills of imagery and awareness. Practice them. Each takes only a few minutes.

How Well Can You Imagine?

The ability to vividly imagine pictures, sounds, feelings, and smells varies widely from person to person. Some people do it with remarkable ease, conjuring images that are clear as the actual event. Others possess varying degrees of ability to imagine ranging from "clear" to "vague." In order to derive benefits from self-hypnosis, you need only to form fairly clear images. Of course, the clearer the image, the better the results you can expect. Do you think you need some help? You can improve your ability to imagine by—you guessed it—practice. Read the following list of items. Pause after each item, close your eyes, and form an image of what you just read. You will notice that some types of images come easier and are much more vivid than others. For instance, colors may be clearer than sounds. Perhaps you can imag-

243

ine a smell more easily than you can imagine a feeling. Doing an exercise such as this is just another way to begin to know yourself better,
to notice how you think, and to make the changes you desire.

Just relax now, and think of:

1. The smell of bread baking in the oven
2. The sounds of an airplane passing overhead
3. The color of your bedroom when you were a child
4. The way ice cream feels in your mouth
5. The sound of a loved one's voice
6. The smile of that same person
7. The feeling of throwing a baseball
8. A stretch of peaceful, sandy beach
9. The sound of popcorn popping
10. The taste of an apple
11. The smell of a rose
12. The warmth of a refreshing shower
13. The feeling of the sheets on your bed
14. The way cooking cabbage smells
15. The feeling of lifting a heavy box
16. Walking up a steep flight of stairs
17. Watching the night sky on an exceptionally clear evening
18. The color of your favorite shirt
19. The sounds of a school playground at recess
20. Walking barefoot on a gravel road

BECOMING "MINDFUL"

Mindful is only another word for awareness, for being awake
and noticing what's going on within you and around you. By now
it will come as no surprise to you that this, too, is a skill that can be
learned and ingrained as a habit. By regularly practicing mindfulness, it will become your usual state. These little exercises will allow
you to monitor your own state of body and mind, and while they

may be a bit uncomfortable in the beginning, the rewards of practice are great. You will come to understand just "how you operate," and this knowledge can be the cornerstone for your self-improvement program. Start to notice the following:

SENSATIONS IN YOUR BODY Focus your attention on your physical body. Watch your breathing rise and fall. Notice sensations such as taste, temperature, muscular tension, color behind your eyelids, feelings of hunger or fullness, and any discomfort you may be experiencing. Can you categorize the sensations as pleasant or unpleasant? Perhaps you just have a neutral feeling. It is natural for the mind to classify information; that's how it always works. When you begin to notice your thoughts, you will probably also begin to notice that they have a life of their own!

SENSATIONS OUTSIDE OF YOUR BODY Observe sensations occurring from an external source such as: the feeling of air moving across your body, the feeling of the chair (or whatever) you're sitting on, the sounds you hear, the source of light you are currently experiencing, and the general feeling of the space you're occupying. Once again, categorize the sensations as pleasant, unpleasant, or neutral.

THE STATE OF YOUR MIND Pay attention to the shifting of your state of mind. Observe how you can, in a very short span of time, feel annoyed, impatient, eager, and peaceful. Categorize these states as you pay attention to them.

OBSERVING YOURSELF Pretend that you are another person, and observe yourself at intervals throughout the day. Make believe that you are across the room and describe what you see. Are you smiling or frowning? Relaxed or tense? Slouching or sitting/standing straight? Alert or tired-looking? By being "outside yourself," you are able to be more honest and objective about what you "see." Do you notice anything you want to change? Now observe yourself by feeling the different parts of your body and describing to yourself how each part feels. Just notice. You don't have to do anything. This exercise is a mini-meditation that you can perform several times each day with your eyes wide open. Give it a try!

Self-Demonstration #1

PENCIL DEMONSTRATION

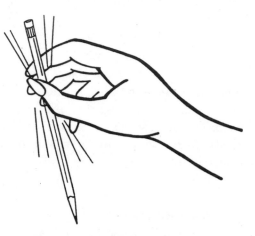

You will need a pencil (or any other object of similar size and shape). Hold it between your thumb and first finger as shown in the illustration. Stare at the pencil intently and say, "I can drop it. I can drop it. I can drop it." Say these words repeatedly with no interruption. During the time you are repeating the sentence over and over in this manner, you can try to drop the pencil, but you will find that you can't. In fact, the harder you try to drop it, the tighter your fingers will grasp it. It is impossible for you to drop the pencil if you are thinking the phrase, as instructed, over and over without interruption. This is a demonstration of the fact that your mind is capable of attending to only one thing at a time and when you are concentrating on the phrase "I can," and not "I am," it is impossible for you to drop the pencil. Change the words to "I am dropping the pencil," or "I drop the pencil," and it happens at once.

Self-Demonstration #2

BOOK AND BALLOON EXPERIMENT

It is important for you to read the instructions completely through before beginning.

Sit comfortably with your feet flat on the floor. Close your eyes and extend your arms from the shoulders straight in front of you, hands up. Close your eyes and imagine: A large, heavy book has been placed on your left hand. In your mind, "see" your hand going down from the weight of the book. "Feel" the book get heavier and heavier as your arm lowers itself with fatigue. Imagine that on your right wrist is a string with a large helium balloon that is rising to the ceiling. As your right hand responds to being "lifted" by the balloon, it seems to drift higher and higher. "Feel" the lightness of your arm as you "see" the balloon take your arm even higher. Imagine the color and size of the balloon. Think of your arm as floating upward. Concentrate for a couple of minutes on the images of the heavy book on your left hand and the balloon on the your right hand. Alternate back and forth between the two images. Then open your eyes. If you have focused on the images as instructed, you will notice that your right arm is higher than the left. The actual distance higher is of no importance. The fact that your imagined "book and balloon" caused a physical reaction is the "proof" that your body carried out the "orders" of your mind.

Self-Demonstration #3

The Pendulum

This is a favorite of ours because the results are so amazing, even mystifying. It is a great exercise to do with a skeptic! You will need a pendulum, or you can construct one from a string or ribbon 12 to 15 inches long with a ring, a washer, or a large button tied to the end for weight.

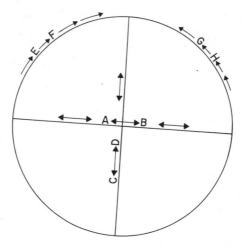

On a plain piece of paper, prepare a visual target as shown in the illustration above. The target is simply a circle that has been divided into 90-degree quadrants by two straight lines intersecting in the center. Designate the lines as A—B and C—D as shown. Designate the clockwise circumference as E—F and the counter-clockwise circumference as G—H. During this experiment, the best position for you to assume is sitting at a desk or a table with your elbow resting on the table. Hold the pendulum string between your thumb and your forefinger as shown in the illustration on the fol-lowing page. Adjust the position of your arm and the way you hold the string so that the bottom of the weight is just touching the cen-ter of the target. Your arm should be at an angle of 45 to 60 degrees to the table top as shown.

Lift the weight barely off the target (1/4"–1/2") and think of movement back and forth along either one of the intersecting lines ("A–B, A–B, A–B" or "C–D, C–D, C–D," etc.). Do not consciously move your hand or the string. Just think on the direction of the line. The pendulum will begin to move in the direction of your thought. Repeat the process with the clockwise and counterclockwise directions.

What really happens here? The pendulum is only amplifying tiny muscles in your wrist and fingers in what is called an ideomotor response. Incidentally, the letters used on the intersecting target and circumference lines can be designated as anything you wish such as "Yes–No," North–South," "Red–Yellow," and the results will be exactly the same.

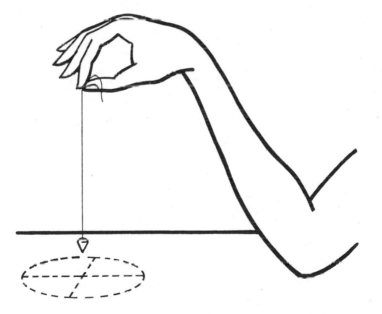

Practicing the Positive

Sometimes we become so accustomed to phrasing things in a negative way that we don't even notice when we're doing it. Your mindfulness practice will enable you to take heed of the words you habitually use on a daily basis. Make it a point to speak only in positive terms in your communication with others. You will be amazed and delighted at the difference in the responses you get! For instance, instead of "Don't forget your jacket," say, "Remember your jacket." Even when you are expressing unhappiness or annoyance, there are ways that make it less hurtful to the other person and more likely to be heard. As we've said before, people cannot make you feel or think anything. Take responsibility for your feelings, and your complaint will make more sense. Here are a few other examples, including some expressions of negative emotions, to help you get the idea:

COMMON PHRASES	ALTERNATIVE PHRASES
Don't get sick.	Be well.
Study or you'll fail.	Study and you'll get a good grade.
You're just driving me crazy.	I get very annoyed at you.
You confuse me.	I don't understand you.
You are so stubborn.	You do have a mind of your own.
If you're not careful, you'll fall.	Hold the rail tightly.

Verbal Vacuuming

The purpose of this exercise is for you to become aware of the clichés and expressions you use. Some of these may be phrases that you have heard and used since childhood, phrases that have become a part of your subconscious beliefs about yourself. Some of them are phrases you use with other people. Notice which of the following are familiar to you. Is there some better way you can express the same thing?

I am:

Burning up

Sick to death of _____

So tired of _____

Worried to death about _____

Torn up over _____

Dead on my feet

Overcome with anxiety

I would die to:

See that

Get that

Have that

Quit work

You are:

Fat

Skinny

A crybaby

A spoiled brat

You'll never get it right.

Other people have it worse than you do.

It's all your fault.

Act your age!

Rich people aren't:

Nice

Spiritual

Honest

Nobody appreciates/understands me.

I have no choice.

I had to eat my words.

I'm such an idiot.

I'm a glutton for punishment.

I can't get it out of my head.

I feel stuffed.

I went berserk.

I almost died.

I'm just a bundle of nerves.

I can't think straight.

I need this like a hole in the head.

I always eat like a pig.

I could just die.

I'm all tied up in knots.

That is a pain in the neck.

I'll have a heart attack.

That tears me apart.

That just makes me sick.

That makes my blood boil over.

That's a tough one to swallow.

That will be the death of me.

I could blow my brains out.

I'll just have to grin and bear it.

I need to have my head examined.

What I don't know can't hurt me.

Verbal vacuuming is a self-explanatory term. It simply means to clean out phrases that you commonly use that may be negatively affecting your life. The purpose of the list is to assist you in noticing the way you conduct your life every day. Your words are indicators of your beliefs. There is an old saying to the effect that an examined life is the life most worth living. Every time you notice yourself thinking or saying phrases that don't enhance your life, just stop. Mentally erase the negative phrase and replace it with a more useful one. Thoughts are habits, too. Make yours work for you!

Self-Hypnosis Therapeutic Suggestions

When you are planning your self-hypnosis session, you will want to pay special attention to the therapeutic suggestions you give to yourself (Step 4 of the 4-A's Method described in Chapter 5). The following suggestions are general, and you should adapt them to your personal situation in whatever way works for you. Use them as they are, or treat them as "springboards" to ideas of your own.

GOAL ACHIEVEMENT SUGGESTIONS:

1. I can do this. I can do whatever I make up my mind to do.
2. I achieve whatever goal I set for myself.
3. I visualize myself succeeding at whatever I choose.
4. This picture of success becomes so strong that it cannot help but become a reality.
5. I do whatever is necessary to succeed.
6. I am already a success. I continue to easily achieve my goals.
7. Every day I list the things I want to accomplish and rank the top priorities.
8. I concentrate on the most important things first.
9. I write down my goals and develop a plan of achieving them.

10. I break down my major goals into monthly, weekly, daily doable mini-goals.

11. Every day I do something to get me closer to my major goals.

12. As I work my goals, I see progress and am motivated to continue.

13. My mind is formulating a plan of what to do and the best way to proceed.

14. I am guided to the persons, situations, knowledge, and help I need.

15. My energy is focused and directed toward my goals.

16. I do the things that guarantee the results I want.

17. I am in charge of my destiny.

18. I do what I need to do to guarantee the future I want.

19. I allow myself to think and dream in unlimited ways.

20. I am born to win! I see myself succeeding in unlimited ways.

TIME MANAGEMENT SUGGESTIONS:

1. My mind is orderly and well organized.

2. I write down what I have to accomplish, prioritize them, and do them in that order.

3. I do what I can, delegate what can be, and let go of the rest.

4. Everything in it's place, and everything in proper proportion.

5. I am calm, confident, and in control of my life and my habits.

6. I ask myself what is the best use of my time and energy now, and I do it.

7. First things first.

8. I rank my tasks by A, B, C, D (delegate), and E (eliminate).

9. I program myself to make the best use of my time.

10. I become better and better organized and efficient, and it is fun. I am punctual.

11. By giving myself extra time, I arrive in a calm, relaxed state of mind.

12. I keep getting better at estimating how long things are going to take.

13. I set realistic, attainable time goals.

14. I use travel time to good advantage.

15. I find ways of combining activities and accomplishing more than one thing at a time.

SELF-ESTEEM SUGGESTIONS:

1. I am worthy of respect, love, prosperity, and success.

2. All good things come to me easily, and I deserve them.

3. My life is valuable.

4. I have many gifts and talents, and I use them well.

5. I am intelligent, practical, and wise.

6. I know what to do and I do it.

7. I am open and receptive to being the best that I can be.

8. I am a good, fair, and honest person of integrity.

9. I like myself.

10. I really enjoy my own company.

11. I am never alone. I always have my best friend with me—me!

12. I let go of my mistakes and focus on who I am and what I have to do right now.

13. I forgive myself and concentrate on what is good about me.

14. I honor and value myself in everything I do.

15. Beauty, love, and balance fill my life. I take time to appreciate what is good about my life, others, and me.

16. I am grateful for all my blessings.

17. All answers are within me.

18. I listen and follow my inner wisdom.

19. I value my time and energy.

20. My path and life's work are my highest priorities.

21. I accept and love myself for who I am right now.

22. I am committed to maximizing my potential.

23. I choose to be alive and grow.

24. I lead a full life.

25. I am enthusiastic and full of zest for life.

26. I am happy and outgoing.

27. My surroundings give me joy and reflect my aliveness and energy.

28. I treat myself lovingly as a treasured friend.

29. I give myself permission to be myself. I give myself permission to laugh, giggle, run, dance, and cry.

30. I release my old ways of behaving.

31. I am willing to change.

32. I release the past.

33. I am free.

34. I am growing and evolving all the time. My awareness daily increases. I exercise appropriate, nonexcessive control over my emotions and behavior.

35. I live totally in the now.

36. I change the past and control the future by changing today.

37. I welcome change.

38. Change is the natural law of life.

39. I move from the old to new ways of thinking and behaving with ease and joy.

40. I am perfect just as I am.

41. I approve of myself.

42. I trust the process of growing and unfolding.

43. I take responsibility for my thoughts, my feelings, and my life.

44. No one and nothing "does" it to me.

45. I am trustworthy, responsible, and dependable.

46. I release all need to make excuses for myself.

47. I do what needs to be done.

48. I am unique.

49. There is no one quite like me.

50. I am discovering new things about me all the time.

51. I have talents and abilities that continuously blossom forth.

52. I am interested in many things.

53. I am always learning and exploring my capabilities and myself.

54. I believe in myself.

55. No one can stop me but me.

56. Rejection is only temporary. It is part of the journey to success.

57. I have a strong belief in myself and in the worth of what I am doing.

58. I am increasingly peaceful and inner-directed.

59. I give generously to myself and give generously of myself to others.

60. I am cheerful and optimistic.

61. I make friends wherever I go.

62. I find something nice to say to my family, co-workers, and people I meet. I look for the good and I find it.

63. I praise others freely and sincerely.

64. Every day I am more patient and understanding.

65. I like being this way!

66. I believe that people are basically good and that life is worthwhile.

67. I demonstrate love with action every day.

68. I release anything and anyone that is not for my highest good.

69. I let go easily, trusting that nothing leaves my life unless something better comes.

70. I bring a positive attitude to everything I do.

71. I am warm and friendly.

72. I only attract people of integrity and goodwill into my life because that is who I am.

73. I value all of my relationships and experiences. I then move on.

74. My intuitive understanding of others increases as I grow in consciousness.

75. I always have a choice.

SUGGESTIONS FOR CAREER DEVELOPMENT:

1. Every day I grow in competence, confidence, and professionalism.

2. I know there is someone looking for just my combination of abilities.

3. I know there is a company looking for exactly what I have to offer.

4. I make a valuable contribution to the place where I work, and I am rewarded.

5. I do what I love with love. Success and money follow.

6. I am always in the right place at the right time.

7. I daily become better at what I do, and it is fun.

8. I am proud of what I have accomplished. I look forward to doing even more.

9. I can make a difference. I have skills and abilities that are needed.

10. I am alert to my opportunities and I use them well.

11. I make a real effort to do my best. I give more and I get more, but first I give.

12. My mind is alert. I listen with interest and absorb rapidly.

13. I speak with authority, conviction, and confidence.

14. Others are interested in what I have to say.

15. My managerial abilities develop rapidly.

16. I focus on being effective—getting the right things done.

17. I have complete poise and confidence in every situation.

18. I make my presentations with showmanship and enthusiasm.

19. I have the initiative and will to succeed.

20. Creativity flows easily wherever it is wanted and needed.

21. I create a wonderful, new job/opportunity now.

22. I always have the most wonderful bosses/clients/customers.

23. My boss/clients/customers always treat me with courtesy and respect.

24. I learn easily and quickly.

25. I remember and call forth information well whenever it is needed.

26. I am always calm, confident, and focused in every test/interview/presentation

27. My work is a joy.

28. I pick and choose the work that is most satisfying to me.

29. I am an irresistible magnet to most wonderful opportunities.

30. I go from success to greater success.

31. I am a success at everything I do.

32. My security is in my worthiness.

33. I have drive, determination, and endurance.

34. Once I know that my course is correct, I stay with it until I succeed.

35. Greatness begins within me.

36. I am always prepared.

37. I do my homework.

38. I give my boss/clients/customers my time and full attention.

39. Every day I grow in ability and visibility.

40. I confront problems with a clear mind and a plan.

SUGGESTIONS FOR PERFORMANCE ANXIETY IN SPORTS AND PUBLIC SPEAKING:

1. I model myself after the best.

2. Every time I hold a club/bat/racket in my hand, I remember the perfect swing and how [mentor] does it.

3. Before I hit the ball, I visualize the ball going exactly where I want it to go.

4. I visualize the perfect outcome/solution/performance before I act.

5. I hear the music played/sung exactly the way I want it before I perform.

6. Perfect mental performance is leading to higher-quality actual performance.

7. Before I make a presentation or speech, I perceive the audience as friendly. I seek to find out what my audience wants and needs and give it to them.

GETTING ALONG WITH OTHERS:

1. I give generously to myself and give generously of myself to others.

2. People like to be with me because I am sincerely interested in them.

3. I listen.

4. I am fun to be around.

5. I see the good in others and help to bring it out.

6. I take time to understand the other person's perspective.

7. I have a real talent for friendship.

8. I make friends wherever I go.

9. I find something nice to say to my family, co-workers, and people I meet.

10. I look for the good and I find it.

11. I praise others freely and sincerely. Every day I am more patient and understanding.

12. I let go of my ego and focus on the spirit of God (truth/love) between us.

13. I believe that people are basically good and that life is worthwhile.

14. I get what I want by giving to others or helping others get what they want.

15. I demonstrate love with action every day.

16. I release anything and anyone that is not for my highest good.

17. I let go easily, trusting that nothing leaves my life unless something better comes.

18. Forgiving feels good.

19. I am too engrossed in living my life to live someone else's life as well.

20. I change the world around me by changing myself.

21. I bring love and a positive attitude to everything I do.

22. I sow love, kindness, consideration, smiles, and service.

23. I get along easily with others.

24. I am warm and friendly.

25. I only attract people of integrity and goodwill into my life because that is who I am.

SUGGESTIONS FOR LOVE RELATIONSHIP:

1. I am a beautiful person.

2. I attract people to me.

3. I know there is a person looking for someone just like me who appreciates me and lovingly accepts me the way I am.

4. I am loving and I am lovable.

5. I am a beautiful (handsome), desirable woman (man) worthy of true love.

6. I listen to the wisdom of my heart.

7. I am open and receptive to true love now.

8. I have a wonderful, mutually supportive relationship now.

9. I deserve the best.

10. Because I love myself, I only attract good relationships into my life.

11. Because I love myself, I groom and dress myself in a careful, loving way.

12. My relationships mirror my relationship with myself.

13. I really enjoy being a man/woman.

14. I am open to myself as a fully functioning sexual being.

15. I love giving of my whole self in a relationship.

16. There is someone good for me.

17. Good relationships are possible, and there is one waiting for me.

18. Like attracts like. I attract nice people because I am one.

19. In all ways I give myself permission to be happy and loved.

20. I deserve to be loved and cherished for the unique person I am.

21. I am being attracted to my ideal mate now.

22. I deserve somebody good.

23. I am ready for a fully committed relationship now.

24. I am open to make new friends.

25. I am open to love again.

26. I meet people worthy of my love and trust.

27. I know that there is someone worthy of my love, trust, and companionship.

28. I recognize and know the right person when he/she comes along.

29. I am perceptive and a wise judge of people.

30. I listen to my intuition and trust my instincts.

31. I know who is good for me.

32. I listen and pay attention to subtle cues.

33. I know my feelings.

34. My mind is clear, as I am a wise, discriminating judge of people.

35. I naturally gravitate to people that are good for me.

36. My choices in a mate are wiser and healthier than ever before.

37. I have the freedom to be me within a committed, loving partnership.

38. I allow others to see who I really am.

39. I allow myself to love deeply and well.

40. I let the other person know how I feel.

41. I set reasonable, healthy boundaries.

42. The only person I can change is me.

43. I do what needs to be done.

44. I take appropriate action.

45. I ask for what I want and need.

References

Ansari, Masud. *Modern Hypnosis: Theory and Practice.* Washington, D.C.: Mas-Press, 1991.

Birkinshaw, E. *Think Slim—Be Slim,* Second Edition. Santa Barbara, Calif.: Woodbridge Press Publishing Co., 1992.

Borysenko, Joan. *Minding the Body, Mending the Mind.* Reading, Mass.: Addison-Wesley Publishing Co., 1987.

Bramwell, J. M. *Hypnotism, Its History, Practice and Theory.* Philadelphia: J. B. Lippincott Co., 1903.

Caprio, Frank S. *Helping Yourself with Psychiatry.* Englewood Cliffs, N.J.: Prentice-Hall, Inc., 1959.

Chopra, Deepak. *Quantum Healing.* New York: Bantam Books, 1990.

Coué, Emile. *How to Practice Suggestion and Autosuggestion.* New York: American Library Service, 1923; Santa Fe, N.M.: Sun Publishing, 1993.

Davidow, Jenny. *Embracing Your Subconscious.* Aptos, Calif.: Tidal Wave Press, 1996.

Elman, Dave. *Hypnotherapy.* Glendora, Calif.: Westwood Publishing, 1984.

Erickson, Milton H., and Linn F. Cooper. *Time Distortion in Hypnosis.* Baltimore: Williams and Wilkins, 1959; New York: Irvington Publishers, 1982.

Estabrooks, G. *Hypnotism.* New York: E. P. Dutton & Co., 1957.

Frankl, Viktor E. *Man's Search for Meaning: An Introduction to Logotherapy.* Boston: Beacon Press, 1992.

Gawain, Shakti. *Creative Visualization.* New York: Bantam Books, 1983.

Hill, Napoleon. *Think and Grow Rich.* Sydney: Angus and Robertson, 1959; New York: Fawcett, 1996.

James, Tad. *The Secret of Creating Your Future.* Honolulu: Advanced Neuro Dynamics, 1995.

James, T., and W. Woodsmall. *Time Line Therapy and the Basis of Personality.* Capitola, Calif.: Meta Publications, Inc., 1988.

265

Krasner, A. M. *The Wizard Within.* Santa Ana, Calif.: ABH Press, 1992.

Kroger, William S. *Clinical and Experimental Hypnosis.* Philadephia: J. B Lippincott Co., 1977.

Levine, Barbara H. *Your Body Believes Every Word You Say.* Boulder Creek, Calif.: Aslan Publishing Co., 1991.

McBrayer, James T. *Hypnotism Simplified.* Baltimore: Mead & Co., 1922.

Maltz, Maxwell, M.D. *Psycho-Cybernetics.* No. Hollywood, Calif.: Wilshire Book Co., 1973.

Ostrander, S., L. Schroeder, and N. Ostrander. *Superlearning 2000.* New York: Dell Publishing, 1994.

Schultz, J. *Autogenic Training.* New York: Grune and Stratton, 1959.

Simonton, O. C. *Getting Well Again.* New York: Bantam Books, 1992.

Spiegel, Herbert, and David Spiegel. *Trance and Treatment.* New York: American Psychiatric Press, Inc., 1987.

Van Pelt, S. J. *Hypnotism and the Power Within.* New York: Fawcett Publications, Inc., 1956.

Virtue, Doreen L. *Constant Craving.* Carson, Calif.: Hay House Publishing, 1994.

——————. *Losing Your Pounds of Pain.* Carson, Calif.: Hay House Publishing, 1994.

Weil, Andrew. *Natural Health, Natural Medicine.* Boston: Houghton Mifflin Co., 1995.

Index

A

Addictions, 112–119
Addictive thinking, 116–117
Aging, 195–200
    See also Longevity
Alcohol abuse, 112–115
    case study, 115–116
    post-hypnotic suggestions, 115
    reasons for, 113
Alcoholics Anonymous, 114
American Board of Hypnotherapy, 221
American Society of Clinical
        Hypnosis, 220
Anger, 154–155
    post-hypnotic suggestions, 155
Ansari, Dr. Masud, relaxation tech-
        nique, 240–242
Attitudes:
    as habits, 139
    changing, 144
    owning, 141–142
Autoanalysis, 74–75, 88
    and depression, 165–166
    of feelings, 142
Autorelaxation, 69–71
Autorelaxation techniques, 225–242
    rapid, 70, 235–236
    clock method, 233–234
    staircase image, 227–230
    tingling sensation, 227–230
Autosuggestion, 32–33, 71–74
Autotherapy, 75–76
    See also Post-hypnotic suggestion

B

Backache, 149
Benefits:
    general, 2–3, 4, 206–207, 210–211
    health, 7, 89–91, 118–119
    self-confidence, 6
    time management, 8–9
    weight loss, 98
Body, functioning of, 35–36, 55
Brain hemispheres, 37–47
    dominance test, 42–47
Brain, 36–50
Bryan, Dr. William J., 201

C

Career development, post-hypnotic
        suggestions, 258–259
Case studies:
    alcohol abuse, 115
    insomnia, 123–124
    sexual dysfunction, 129, 130–131
    smoking, 109–112
    tension, 137–139
    weight loss, 96–97, 99–102
Childhood, conditioning in, 26
Children and hypnosis, 218
Cigarette smoke, chemical makeup,
        106
Claustrophobia, 156–157
Color, use in pain control, 149
Concentration, 185
Conditioned response, 28–31

Conditioning:
    habits, 28
    in childhood, 26
Conscious mind, 52–54
Corpus callosum, 37
Coué, Emile, 32
Creativity, 5, 38, 41

D

Daily planning, 84–86
Decision-making, 54
Depression, *See* Mental depression
Dieting, 91, 93, 94
    See also Weight control
Direct suggestions, 24
Dominant brain hemispheres, 37–47
Dreams, 58–59
Drinking problem, *See* Alcohol abuse
Drug addiction, 116–119
    post-hypnotic suggestions, 118–119
    symptoms, 116
Drug therapy, 4

E

Eating habits, 92–96
    See also Weight control
Ego, 173
Emergencies, 76–77
Emotion:
    and fear, 153
    and habits, 29
Emotional problems, 77–78
    and eating, 93–94, 102
    and sexual dysfunction, 127
    depression, 165–171
Endocrine deficiency, 196
Enjoyment, planning for, 86, 91
Erickson, Dr. Milton, 3–4
Escape mechanisms, 113
Exercises:
    for sleep, 125–126
    imagery, 243–244
    positive thinking, 250–252

visualization, 48–49
    See also Mind exercises
Eye closure test, 71

F

Fatigue, 122
    and boredom, 199–200
    and sexual problems, 128
    and tension, 140–141
Fear:
    and emotion, 62–63, 151–163
    and negative emotion, post-hypnotic
        suggestions, 153–155, 161–163
    of failure, sexual, 131, 133
    of flying, 159–163
Feelings, changing, 144
4-A's method, 69–76
Freud, Sigmund, 13
Frigidity, 128–129
Frustration, 60–62

G

Goals:
    achievement of, 186–187
    and motivation, 57
    attainment of, 76
    listing, 84–85
    post-hypnotic suggestions, 253–254
    setting, 64–66
Grief, overcoming, 197–199
Guilt, 153–154
    and sleeplessness, 124

H

Habits, 89
    formation.of, 107
    forming, 28–29
    smoking, 105–110
Hand-tingling test, 73
Happiness:
    and love, 9, 19–20
    formula for, 209

Headache, 148
Health risks:
   cigarettes, 105
   obesity, 92
Health-wisdom, 89
Healthy lifestyle, 89–91, 118–119
   daily reminders, 90–91
Hereditary predispositions, 207
Hollander, Dr. Bernard, 19–20
Humor, 145
Hypnosis defined, 12–13
Hypnotherapist, professional, 220–221
Hypnotic equivalents, 191–192
Hypnotic state, demonstrations of,
   246–249

I

Imagery, exercises to improve,
   243–244
Impotence, 131–132
Impulses, 54–55
Indirect suggestions, 24
Information processing, 52–54
Inherited traits, 207
Inhibitions, release from, 113–114
Inner self, 6
Insomnia, 121–123
   See also Sleep, Sleeplessness
Interpersonal relationships, 179,
   189–194
   post-hypnotic suggestions, 260–261
   See also Relationships
Interruptions, 77, 215
Intuition, 38, 40, 41

J

James, Dr. Tad, 64–66

K

Key words, relaxation, 70

L

Laughter, to reduce tension, 145
Lazarus, Dr. Arnold, 47
Learning ability, 183–185
   case study, 185–186
Left-brain functions, 37–41, 52
Length of sessions, 213–214
Linear thinking, 41
Listening skills, 178
Listing goals, 84
Location of sessions, 213, 218
Logical reasoning, 37
Longevity, 195–200
   case study, 197–199
   endocrine deficiency, 196
   post-hypnotic suggestions, 204
   will to live, 196–197
Love relationships, 9, 19–20, 127,
   134–135
   See also Relationships
Love, of self, 128

M

Magnetic personality, 178
Measurable goals, 64
Media influence, body weight, 92–93
Medical diagnosis, 77, 205
   depression, 167
   pain, 146
Memory, 53–54, 55, 183–184
Mental depression, 165–171
   case studies, 168–170
   post-hypnotic suggestions, 171
Mind exercises
   awareness, 244–245
   mental harmony, 48–49
   imagery, 243–244
Mind, conscious and subconscious,
   51–56, 206
Misconceptions, 14–18, 205, 219
Moodiness, 165–166
Motivation, 57
   for habit-breaking, 108
Music, in autorelaxation, 69

N

Negativity:
  attitudes, 161
  emotions, 153
  images, 81
  suggestions, 30
  words, 251–252

O

Obesity, 92
Occupational stress, 140–141
  See also Tension
Organization, and time management,
  8–9

P

Pain, 53, 145–150
  and sleeplessness, 122
  imagery, 148–149
  post-hypnotic suggestions, 149–150
Past suggestions:
  and food, 92–93
  power of, 81
Pavlov, Dr. Ivan, 28–29
Performance anxiety, post-hypnotic
  suggestions, 260
Personality:
  assessing flaws, 68, 74–75
  development, 7–8, 26, 173–174
  case study, 181–183
  changes in, 175–179
  components of, 175
  factor in success, 190
  self-defeating, 176
Phobia, *See* Fear
Physical disease, and depression, 167
Placebos, 216
Planning, 8–9
  advantages of, 86
  for self-improvement, 83–88
  making lists, 84–85
Positive conditioning, 31

Positive thinking, 6, 75–76, 144,
  169–170
  as religion, 202
  practice exercises, 250–252
Post-hypnotic suggestions:
  addiction, 118–119
  additional lists, 252–263
  alcohol abuse, 115
  interpersonal relationships,
    179–180
  longevity, 204
  memory improvement, 184
  mental depression, 171
  pain control, 149–150
  power and appeal, 194
  reinforcement, 212
  sales success, 192–193
  sexual problems, 130, 134–135
  sleep disorders, 123–124
  smoking, 108–109, 111–112
  timing of, 73–74
  tolerance, 180–181
  weight-loss, 94–96
  worry, 144
Power over others, 189–194
Practice, benefit of, 79
Prayer, 201
Problem-solving, overnight, 59–60
Psychological suicide, 92, 113
Psychosomatic illness, 7, 51
  and tension, 140

R

Rapid relaxation, 70
Realistic goals, 65
Recreation, 91
Rejuvenation, 195
Relationships, 9, 179, 189–194
  love, 261–263
  and sex, 127, 134–135
Relaxation, *See* Autorelaxation
Relaxation, pharmaceutical, 4
Religion, 201–203
Religious belief, 203

Resistance, to hypnotic suggestion,
    15–16
Response, conditioned, 28–29
Right-brain functions, 37–41, 52
Ripple effect, 80
Root conflict, 58
Rousing from hypnosis, 76

S

Sabotage, 80
Sales ability, 191–193
Self-analysis, 68, 74–75
    of feelings, 142
    of sexual problems, 129, 132, 134
    See also Autoanalysis
Self-confidence, 6, 86, 191
Self-destruction, 92, 113
Self-discipline, 8–9
Self-esteem, 191
    post-hypnotic suggestions, 255–258
Self-fulfilling prophecies, 62
Self-improvement, making a plan,
    83–88
Self-mastery, 51, 208
Self-relaxation, *See* Autorelaxation
Self-suggestions, word choice, 63–66
Sexual problems, 127–135
    post-hypnotic suggestions, 130,
        134–135
    self analysis, 129, 132, 134
    sexual response, 128–129, 135
Shyness, 182
Simonton, Dr. Carl, 140
Sleep, 16, 121
    and problem-solving, 59–60
    during trance, 217–218
Sleeplessness:
    reasons for, 122–123, 124
    remedies, 125
S.M.A.R.T. goals, 64–66
Smoking, 105–112
    case studies, 109–112
    conditioned response, 28–29
    dangers of, 105–106

Social isolation, 168–169, 181–182
Spiegel's relaxation technique,
    241–242
Stage fright, 157
    post-hypnotic suggestions, 260
Staircase technique, 227–230
Stress, *See* Tension
Subconscious mind, 52–53, 54–56
    access to, 56
    and personality, 174
    controlling functions, 55
    creativity, 56
    dreams, 59
Success, sales occupations, 191–193
Suggestibility, 12–13, 16, 23, 24–26,
    71, 206
    tests for, 71–73
Suggestions:
    negative, 30
    post-hypnotic, 73–74
    receiving, 24–26
    repeated, 92–93
Swallowing test, 72

T

Technique, 69–76, 225–242
Tension, 137–146
    and fatigue, 140–141
    as a habit, 139–140
    case study, 137–139
    sexual, 128
    work-related, 141
Tests of hypnotic state, 71–73
Theory, nature of hypnosis, 13
Time management, 8–9
    post-hypnotic suggestions, 254–255
Tolerance, 180
Trance state:
    deepening, 216–217
    recognizing, 214–215
    sleeping, 217–218
Transference, 13, 179
Treatments for alcoholism, 114
Treiber, Ken, 209–210

U

Unhappiness, 165–171
    See also Mental depression

V

Visual suggestions, 193–194
Visualization:
    exercises, 48–49
    and fear of flying, 161
    and pain control, 148–149

W

Waking from hypnosis, 76
Waking state, relaxation in, 70
Weight control, 91–103
    benefits, 98
    case studies, 96–97, 99–102
    dieting, 91, 93, 94
    emotional issues, 93–94
    motivations, 95
    nine-step program, 94–96
    obesity, 92
Willpower, 103
Words, in self-suggestions, 63–64
Words, negative, 66, 251–252
Work stress, contributes to smoking,
        111
Worry, 143–144
    insomnia, 122
    as acquired habit, 143
    post-hypnotic suggestions, 144
Written plans, 84–85